THE DOS AND DON'TS OF MANAGING CARERS

A Guide To Efficient And Compassionate Care For
Care Home Managers And Government Agencies

CH'KA AMAECHI

First published in paperback and kindle in 2020
Publisher: Independently published
Language: English
ISBN: 9798692403575
Imprint: Independently published

This non-fiction book is based on observations and experiences of the author. To maintain confidentiality and protect the privacy, names of people and venue have been excluded except in situations where such names or venues were already in the publicly accessed publications. Any other similarities are purely coincidental.

Table of Contents

Introduction

Shall I begin by paraphrasing Chinua Achebe's words; if you do not like my story, simply write your own.

The fact that most UK care homes are run by their shareholders solely on a commercially-driven terms is a bad thing and the entire country has indeed abandoned their responsibilities of looking after their elderly in not-for-profit basis in the same way that basic education for children should be free and non-profit oriented. Due to this privatised pro-profit approach, prolonged underfunding by the 2010s succeeding Thatcherite UK governments and shareholders and in some cases failure of Care Homes' management to proactively implement best practices of Human Resource Management, there have been significant shortcomings in the quality of care in the UK adult social care. It is nothing but a profound sense of sentimental naivety to expect excellent quality of care services with the current situation. There is a limit which regulation of the industry can go to maintain standard and there is also a limit which the unsung heroes of the industry can be stretched.

This memoir aims to share stories of challenges, explore basic problem-solving skills subconsciously developed and guide all stakeholders on how to handle the care industry's complex issue with regards to creating a genuinely compassionate environment and providing effective service.

This memoir aims to guide managers on how to promote compassionate care in their care homes in line with the laws of compassion which cannot be legislated out of existence. This memoir takes a stance: For a care home to truly be compassionate, it must begin by showing compassion to its employees. If a care home cannot offer its own employees an understanding, forgiveness and loving kindness, that care home can never give genuine compassion to its residents.

This memoir highlights the critical and the reality of the private care industry in the UK at this time based on the sole perspective of the writer, such first-hand witnessed problems as were compounded by the extreme underfunding by the UK government. Each new year ushers in a new record low and an accelerated standard decline and compromises that are traceable to underfunding and profit-oriented industry. These are tough, desperate and challenging times for local authorities dealing with cuts & difficult decisions, families, residents and Carers. We are all in it together. This memoir is advocating that families see Carers as partners on the same forefront rather than people to take frustrations out on.

This memoir is in no way defending any form of abuse or malpractice, rather this memoir focuses on tracing and highlighting the underlying & possible sources of most mistakes, neglects and abuses in Care Homes in order to find sustainable approaches and ways of eradicating abuse by cutting it far beneath the root level. The writer suggests ways of alleviating some of the problems. This memoir will advocate provision of profound support for Carers in events of mistakes especially Carers working long hours in pressured environments instead of the callous scapegoat of one Carer or care home that has made a mistake for failures in the system as by so doing discourage Carers from being open to their managers or other safeguarding authorities when reviewing mistakes or shortcomings.

Any assertion made in this memoir should be understood to be based on facts as kept from January 2013 to the published date during which the writer has worked in failing, failed, struggling and successful award-winning care homes as a frontline care staff and has accrued a great deal of knowledge and first-hand experience. With his previous Masters level academic experience, he is able to give, good analysis, advice relating to adoption and implementation of best practice human resource management by care homes management as well as advice on how relatives could get involved in order to help a struggling and underfunded public and private health care industry of the United Kingdom.

This memoir will pay attention to detail, but the writer will try to summarise as much as possible since the aim is to deliver the message at quickest reading-time possible.

This memoir is intended to provide a general guide to the various issues discussed. Specialist advice should be sought about your specific circumstances.

Finally, this memoir aims solely to point out the wrongs, how to correct them and promote the good in adult social care; hence, should not by no means portray the writer as a very vain, self-important and pompous ass who pretends he knows everything.

Terminologies as used specifically in this book
Carers
A carer is an individual who is employed to look after the elderly in nursing or residential home or in the elderly person's own home. The word, 'carers' may be substituted for, 'care workers' or 'staff'.

Residents
A resident is an elderly individual or younger person who lives in a residential or nursing home of the elderly and receive care no matter what degree of care being received. The word, 'residents' may be substituted for, 'service users'.

Relatives
A relative is an individual whose loved one(s) lives and receive care in a residential or nursing home.

Care Homes
A Care home is a generalised word for either a nursing or residential home.

Residential Homes
A residential home is a care home where residents does not require the services of a live-in nurse. They are mostly able to cater for themselves to a considerable extent.

Nursing Homes
A nursing home is a care home which have a live-in nurse every hour of the year and residents' needs are mostly advanced hence the need for nursing care.

Investors
An Investor is the owner or part-owner or director or shareholders of the care home business who earns the profits or bears the loss.

Managers
A manager is an individual who is employed by the Investors to manage the care home on their behalf.

Government Agencies
Government agencies are all organs of the government that regulates or manages the wider social care sector on behalf of the government. They include the CQC (Care Quality Commission), Local Safeguarding team, ENRICH team (Enabling Research in Care Homes) NHS (National Health Service), PHE (Public Health England) and the DHSC (Department of Health and Social Care).

Management

Care business strategy

Based on experience, the underlying reasons behind failed care homes can usually be traced to a bad strategy. Care is an aspect of the healthcare industry that requires seriously deciding what you do and what you do not do and stringently sticking to your strategic decision.

When a care home wants to be simultaneously running an assessment unit, nursing and residential in the same premises; that is a bad strategy in most places that I have been. Very ambiguous and Jack of all trade philosophy.

In one residents meeting that I attended, few residential residents' complaints were related to them not having peaceful life because the nursing residents disturb and take all the attention while they themselves become neglected and at the same time the nursing residents don't let them have peaceful dining at mealtimes and lounge relaxation is never without verbal related disturbances. If allowed to occur for a while, your residential residents may leave the care home due to the above issues. Assessment unit is a unit for assessment of individuals who have never been in care ever before and are to be assessed with a view of them returning home after hospital admission. The problem with mixing this unit is because in all the places I have seen it being run side by side with a residential home, they often fail to distinguish it as initially planned and you end up not running it as its own unit independent and self-catering. The home manager often disregards that the advantage care homes have which is that back-of-hand knowledge of its residents by Carers. A Carer may return from a 3 weeks holiday abroad and perform as if she or he has not even left for a day because she already knows all the residents too well.

My little nephew, a toddler, tries to speak to me but I did not hear or understand a single word of his. He turned around and spoke to his parents and they understood everything that he said. So, I asked how you understood him, and they chuckled and said to me that they have been understanding him from when he was a baby and could not talk, and now his gibberish language makes more sense. In a nutshell, they really know him because they are his parents. This is another good instance of my point. But when you bring in residents in the assessment unit, their needs are unknown so as their names and character. That is why they need close and special monitoring which cannot be achieved by combining their unit and its special needs with your other already assessed residents. I recall an evening when I arrived to work a night shift and saw many doctors from the NHS walking about. I was told that a 92-year-old lady was discharged from the hospital into our assessment unit which ran side by side with our care home. One of us was asked to go and stay in the assessment unit for the night. The hospital did not inform us that they knew the newly admitted lady was at the end of her life and we did not know much about her. In the early hours of that first night in our assessment unit, we had to be monitoring her closely as we found her breathing very bad and knew that a serious situation had fallen on our hands. She stopped breathing while we were talking to the hospital on the phone, the paramedics arrived immediately and took over the resuscitation. The other paramedic administered a medication via her shoulder bone, continuing CPR as we heard her ribs cracking and the other paramedic began to read her medical history and questioned why has a lady with all these issues not have a DNAR (do not attempt cardiopulmonary resuscitation) in place and response was, she was just admitted the previous evening from the hospital into the home's assessment unit and we actually only getting to know her.

The real situation is that this lady was discharged in line with the hospital's cynical move to avoid people dying in their care and discharging them just before they die but this lady cannot be discharged back to her house so they sent her to an assessment unit but did not inform the staff detailed issues about her or if they did, such detail weren't effectively passed on to us and that is totally bad.

On the other hand, having residents with advanced dementia (nursing) live with other residents who have only just moved into the care home affects the overall wellbeing of the later residents. They will get lesser attention.

Quality or quantity

If you have a less than 20 room house to be used for a care home, then you are better off transforming it to the best quality care home that gives most personalised care in the UK. Raise your weekly fee and allow room sharing. set the pace and let others learn from you. Win all winnable awards for excellence. And relatives would be willing to pay the higher rate. You represent the future because personally since classrooms are restricted to 30 pupils according to policy administered by the Education Authority, then care homes must be sooner or later restricted to not more than 35 residents. These 60-bed homes should be closed.

Volunteer, become a Carer for a day

All stakeholders in the care industry, especially relatives, directors, and managers should volunteer to work with Carers twice each year one night and one day shift. This is an essential need.

Clear instructions and Kaizen

The sort of issues management fails often to understand which this memoir aims to highlight are very simple and plain common-sense issues in whatever way they are looked at. Take, for instance, managers require Carers to write and record a great deal of information. Write this, fill that form, record and so on but they will not provide any writing pen. The pen is mightier than the sword only if the pen is provided. "If it is not written, it didn't happen" is a sign posted on most Carers' notice board, only for the pen to remain unavailable. It is important for management to get first-hand experience of the job in order to manage Carers and other staff.

The management style of a care home is mostly about operation and efficiency. A care home should be a learning organisation and managers must be able to deliver clearly defined instructions to well-trained but uneducated staff. A clearly defined instruction also considers time-budgeting in line with all tasks that are required to be attended to into consideration as well as unknown tasks that may emerge out of nowhere. Avoid ambiguous objectives. Ambiguity leads to lying. As simple as that based on what I have observed. When a manager gives instructions, it must be feasible and without any over-ambitious or ambiguous objectives. If you want Carers to do 15 minutes interval observation on a resident in her bedroom for instance, you must first realise that it is more than just popping your head into the room and out as there is paperwork to complete and few minutes required to interact with that resident and you must ensure that it is indeed feasible in terms of staffing levels, other tasks that the Carers had been given and time. This sort of check is almost equal to designating one member of the team to do no other job but observe this 15 minutes interval check and document it because walking to the bedroom takes some minutes, the check itself takes some minutes, documenting the check takes some minutes, walking back to continue what the Carer was doing before the check takes some minutes. If this person also has lots of other things to do, then if she is assisting someone else with personal care, can one of her teammates be able to pause whatever she is doing in order to observe the 15 minutes interval room check? If Carers see the ambiguity in the instructions and they won't challenge your instructions, then they will fill in the 15 minutes observation form records detailed for you as if it had been observed up to your instructed extent but the truth remains that the ambiguity killed their moral and they cowardly gave you what you want to see. This is very prevalent in care homes and that is why it should be fixed. Being reasonable requires any manager to ask Carers if they can or if they need additional staff. Poor time budgeting and planning leads to stress and Carers rushing to satisfy huge demands and they simply cannot hide the adrenaline and body language from such feelings and stress. Residents feeling rushed emanate usually from this uncontrollable body language of Carers who are rushed. When a Carer is given a list of 10 residents to assist with washing and dressing and assisting to the dining table to eat breakfast. That Carer has from the time the Carer's handover ends (assume 7:30am) to the maximum reasonable time for eating breakfast. Take, for instance, a resident whose physiotherapist recommended walking some distance in the morning, the Carers after getting her washed and dressed would walk with her from the bedroom to the dining room. Due to the resident's slow walking pace it will take extra 10/15 minutes but then the Carers don't have that time and as a matter of fact, this time wasn't budgeted at all and now add this unbudgeted time to the other requirement to observe a 15 minutes interval room check on another resident.

Because it was ambitious and ambiguously designed gets every Carer to apparently subconsciously involved in disobeying instructions and for the Same reason, the entire whistleblowing policy collapses and even the most dedicated Carer who will accept nothing but best quality care becomes useless, frustrated and complacent. A very good example is the ' hourly night turns and checks' which means that every hour, a resident's sleep is disturbed and at some point, all Carers would subconsciously agree that it is unfair to the resident and therefore to falsify that it is actually done hourly and rather, they may do the checks on hourly basis quietly but not do the turn hourly but they will write that the resident was turned hourly. The hourly repositioning of residents at this particular care home that I worked was only changed to bi-hourly after the manager had to come in and work with me because she reduced the staffing level from 3 Carers and a nurse down to 2 Carers and a nurse and one night when I was working, a Carer had to go home to take her sick son to the hospital in the middle of the night and third party recruitment agencies could not find a replacement. The manager came in and worked with me and the nurse from around midnight and realised that the hourly repositioning rate was ambiguous in an actual sense. We could not even complete one round of repositioning residents in an hour before restarting the round all over again. The manager was kept on her feet throughout the night and she realised that none of the domestic duties such as cleaning and laundry could be done. By morning, she extended the hourly repositioning to two-hourly.

Another good example is the 15 minutes observations where Carers are instructed to check a resident every 15 minutes. It is just impossible at rush hour times hence they falsify that it was done.

Signs of Failing

Staff retention is the watchword and yardstick for measuring healthy your care home is. Experience has shown me that Care home first loses its best staff before closing or shutting down. The staff usually get fed up with not being heard as well as a series of issues with the home and quietly leave one by one. That is the best warning of imminent doom.

Other signs may include several trails of safeguarding issues and complaints, getting in and out of barred admission by the local council. These are a series of occurrences that happen before closure or withdrawal of council-funded residents from a home.

Understaffing: Stop! Whipping running horses

We see jockeys whip their horses in a bid to make the horse run faster even though the horse is already running at its own maximum speed at that time. This is exactly what is happening now in each understaffed shift in care homes. Understaffing has consequences. Its greatest consequences are the plunge in standards, especially safety (of residents and Carers). The problem with understaffing is that Carers get blamed or threatened for these consequences of understaffing. Let us look at this particular text message, "All staff- nobody should ever reposition or turn alone. If it comes to light that anyone does this, you will face instant disciplinary action against you". This text is referring to any Carer who risks injury to his/herself to get residents repositioned as required by him/herself when that task requires two Carers. It is usually caused when Carers are overburdened and overstretched making them work like that in order to finish on time specially to avoid being cautioned against not completing the huge tasks assigned to them before going home. The management should instead of sending this sort of text (threat), reassess why Carers were struggling. It is a very clear 'over-speeding' and can potentially make Carers work individually when they are supposed to work in twos. It can also make Carers work in twos but in a very ridiculously fast manner which is equally dangerous and generally plunges quality of care. The other consequence of understaffing is the tendency to get residents up in very early/late hours in the morning or get residents into bed far too early or late in the evening. Too often the CQC visits care homes at 6am in the morning and found many residents who had already been assisted up sitting and sleeping in the lounges. CQC questioned why they were not sleeping in their respective bedrooms and no one could answer that. The management would eventually blame the Carers for it but there are many pressures from the management which make Carers engage in such institutional abuse. Such pressures to do more include the following sort of text message from the management to the night staff, "Hi all if M asks for a shower at 4.30am you shower her you do not say it's too early. No matter what time it is if she asks for a shower you must do it. Also, you need to be doing more bed baths for the main house, not just the extension.

Thanks". It is such pressure to help make it easier for the understaffed morning team which the management will later deny. Look closely at the text and notice that the management simply said get more residents up by saying that they need to be doing more bed baths but did not care about whether the residents wish to get up that early.

But why must Carers bear the consequences when they did not cause the understaffing in the first place. A good example of the consequence can be seen when a resident falls down due to low response time caused by understaffing (Carers genuinely being busy with other residents who themselves are at falls risk so cannot be left alone in other for the overstretched Carer leave to respond quickly to another falls risk resident), the management in a bid to show on record that some preventive measures are in place to stop recurrence, they put 15 minutes intervals check on such residents that have fallen thereby giving more work to already overwhelmed care staff. Furthermore, instead of adding more staff, they arrange falls prevention training mandating Carers to attend thereby preventing Carers from enjoying their days off. And falls would remain imminent. If there are ten residents in a home who are highly likely to fall if any of them attempt to stand up and walk, and there are three Carers on shift, how safe are the residents? CQC and local authorities should stop grading staffing levels based on a few staff in each shift without having a good look at the need and risk of falls of each resident living in that care home.

Staffing ratio
Use of staffing ratio to ascertain the number of staff needed for each shift based on the number of residents is bad and the right thing is to Base staffing levels on the needs of the residents. The biggest problem in care today is some residents are significantly at risk of hurting themselves or another resident on a 24 hours basis and therefore passes for 'one to one' monitoring which is very expensive. As of now, it appears easier to pass a camel through a needle hole than to get 'one to one' funding for a resident literally. But staffing issues have very little to do with local authorities, it has a lot to do with profit margin and end of year bonuses of high-ranking management. The fact that care homes are profit-making ventures mean that profit margin involved the manager to proactively adopt policies aimed at reducing operation and running cost daily. When a kitchen staff phone-in sick, squeeze a Carer from the care team to man the kitchen post and let them Carers manage anyhow. But this issue

is not limited to care homes, the NHS was forced to review the bills for using agency staff to cover shifts. Agency covers are expensive but necessary.

No time is usually budgeted for wandering residents with extreme anxiety and risk of falls who aren't on one-to-one scheme, a situation which demands that a Carer must urgently be designated to wander with that particular resident as close as possible and must prevent the resident from falling or opening other residents doors to walk into their room and disturb their sleep or peace and at the same time attend to the call bells. Carer would be pointing out to the resident who is walking unsteadily about how unsteady he/she is and how dangerous it is but to actually force the resident to sit or remain seated is not permitted and classed as abuse (physical abuse). To give up on the resident and let him/her disturb others, or fall since he/she is not listening is also not permitted and regarded as abuse (neglect) should a fall happen and the Carer is expected to walk/wander along with the resident. This expectation contravenes with moving and handling training advice to never attempt to catch any resident that is falling so, therefore, the expectation is not to catch rather, to help a resident remain/maintain regular balance as he/she wanders about. Too many falls occurring in any care home is deemed to be due to neglect by external stakeholders while internally it is blamed on Carers slow response time but the reality remains that Carers are overloaded with tasks and no time is budgeted for this particular sort of fall prevention assistance. A certain abuse that led to Carers being imprisoned for tying a resident to a chair and locking up a resident is a good instance of symptoms of this failure to adequately allocate/budget time for this issue.

No time is usually budgeted for residents in respective bedrooms who just hate being alone or feel frightened or anxious or use the toilet frequently due to prostate related issues or for any other reason seeks attention and persistently uses the call bell to ring over and over or stands on the floor sensor mat over and over. This means constantly dashing to this sort of resident and could sometimes prevent Carers from doing several other things that they must do before the next shift commences. A Carer is usually told off for answering a call bell in a visibly stressed up & frustrated mood. It is, in fact, an on-the-spot dismissal offence.

No time is usually budgeted for residents who need feeding and the fact that such residents often eat slowly due to choking risks. In some care homes, a Carer must feed a few other people and must finish assisting one person in order to move on to the next person. In one care home, CQC agents caught a Carer feeding two people at the same time. The Carer shed tears when she heard gossips blaming her for the poor CQC report.

I read someone describe depression as walking through deep snow while at the same time you can see other people ice skating around. Having said that, why will not the best Carers leave their adult social care jobs for other industries like retails, security, manufacturing or even support workers for learning disability residents.

Staff moaning at each other
Take, for instance, night staff are expected to do laundry washing hanging ironing, mopping, hovering, cleaning & wiping, peeling potatoes, cutting vegetables, setting dining tables, getting cups and bowls out of kitchen cupboards and putting them at the kitchen island /serving desk bar. The Carers do these as well as their main job of looking after residents.

The most prevalent of the problems are Carers are moaned at by the main kitchen cooks and the main domestic workers if one of these is not done up to their expected standards. They often do not care whether the night Carers were busy all night or not, whether they were well trained or taught to do these duties especially newly employed Carers. The fact that night staff have been up all night and other staff moan at them in the morning are terrible. The manager must ensure this never even happens in the first place. Must always remind the kitchen team and other domestic staff that since they would not be expected to be perfect Carers, and they will not be given care responsibilities, then they should stop expecting perfection from the Carers when they help out with kitchen and other domestic duties which are not their own main duties and responsibilities. The sort of grievance and hurt feelings this sort of issue causes lingers sometimes for the entirety of the employment. As a matter of fact, in some care homes, kitchen and domestic staff always have a notorious member of their team 'hated' by some care staff and I use that word 'hated' because it is the right word that qualifies what I have seen.

When a care home recruits new Carers, there is that tendency of the incoming newbie to please the manager by doing more work, more stress. In many cases, this goes further to snitching/spying on teammates by informing the manager of whatever happens in the shift, every gossip, who said this, who said that. The impact of this act destroys the team beyond repair, so it is in the Management's interest to discourage it. The little benefit of having an ear listening in on your staff does not outweigh the problem of having some Carers leave their job as a result of collapse in teamwork or professional relationships.

Vertical correction communications only

The manager should during induction or staff meetings and at staff notice boards highlight that all dissatisfied/moaning or complaints must be made vertically to the manager's office and all threats of disciplinary action or warnings or corrective actions that are to be made to any member of the staff team must only come directly from the manager's office and no staff should verbally or by any other means warn or threaten other staff, warn another staff or impose corrective measures on other staff. This is not for Carers alone; relatives and residents should make their regular complaints to the management directly.

Please dear colleague, do not boss me about

The care environment is a fast moving, developing environment very stressful in nature. staff feel more pressured when they are not allowed to use their own initiatives and whenever they are doing something, another staff will interfere to supervise and tell them what they already know. When they set out to do a task in room A, another staff will call them back halfway into the walk toward room A only to inform them to go to room A and do the exact same thing they initially set out to go and do. This brings a heightened level of stress into an already stressful situation. I was working on this care home, right after breakfast, I began to remove dirty tablecloths, the bossy colleague then shouted from a distance, don't remove the table clothes, I didn't hear her so I responded 'what did you say' she repeated, 'don't Change the table clothes unless they are dirty'. I wondered if there is anywhere in my face where it is written that I am stupid and that I needed regular supervision with changing table clothes. Bossy staff think there is a need for them to help with delegating jobs to other staff of equal level and status, but such need is for the senior or manager of higher level and status to fill. I have only included this in this memoir so that managers know what a staff member is talking about when they say someone is bossing them about.

Eye-service is not any staff's duty

In earlier chapters, I described certain staff members who you usually see keeping a visiting-relative company when they visit even though there are numerous reasons to be elsewhere where duties were called. These sorts of staff are prone to breaching confidentiality agreements knowingly or unknowingly because relatives often ask confidential questions about other care home residents and their medical or mental health conditions and these mentioned staff tend to disclose the information. They sometimes use this opportunity to talk bad about their fellow staff and sometimes about the home itself just to appear to be well 'liked' by visiting relatives. As soon as a relative arrives, that is when they start looking after the relative's resident in a helter-skelter or over-committed sort of manner. They would spend a great deal of time in the office discussing with the manager or team leader, oh yes, they are good companions but at the end, the manager questions why jobs are not completed. They also use this closeness to a manager or team leader to influence their judgement and indulge in performance defamation of their colleagues.

These sorts of Carers specialise in delegating tasks to newer members of staff or staff on zero-hour contracts or from recruitment agencies as opposed to doing the task. Avoid this sort of worker like a plague. They destroy teams and make a mockery of the word 'diligence' or say working hard. Most of all, their attitude to work puts more stress and pressure on their teammates who will have to do more or else nothing will be done. Their attitude and laziness kill the morale of everyone else. Worse is, they will never be reported by other staff should they do something bad because they are a manager or team leader's best friend. The advantage of having this 'best friend' who acts as the manager's spy who keeps him or her well informed about every staff's actions both in and outside work or makes sure that managers tea or coffee cups never go dry is lost when the same spy influences your judgement by telling lies or exaggerating facts plus the fact that the manager cannot be viewed as a fair or reliable judge on any dispute involving staff.

Managers should detect this happening and avoid getting too attached to these sorts of Carers. Remind them to leave your office and do some work or remind them that you are the manager and do not need any escort within your office or during your cigarette breaks or someone to help you analyse data or spy on staff. I have seen situations where managers promote this attitude to work. I'm talking about situations where the manager and that sort of staff get too close and would sit down in the office regularly having a chat or even where manager or team leader would ask a staff member who isn't on his or her break to accompany the manager or team leader to go out for a cigarette, sometimes this could happen bi-hourly totally ignoring the burden this would place on staff who are also working. Time lost can never be recovered, unanswered call bells plus duties which are not done yet must be done by someone else as they pile up. Other staff will be stressed, not be happy and cannot speak up, as this happens, their compassion for the job suffers and the quality of care drops.

One manager did something incredible, one Carer who had this behaviour and could not be sacked was asked to become the activities coordinator which is far removed from the busy part of the team.

Using listed buildings

These very old buildings were not designed to serve this purpose. Converting them into care homes present lots of challenges. For example, in all such buildings, the buildings are too hot in summer because windows are impossible to open for fresh air because they are too delicate or there is always something wrong and single glazed so it is too cold in winter. They should be avoided and if it must be used, then there should be a standard that must be met. A situation where the Hoist cannot get to every room or lots of steps or windows not opening/ shutting completely or high risk of asbestos or legionnaires disease. In the Summer, the bees fly into the building from the only openable window and get trapped and every morning you see over 100 bees and wasp were dead on the floor near the other non-opening windows.

Efficiency

Inefficient daily duty allocation

It is very good to allocate duties and responsibilities to each member of your care staff to trace completions or otherwise badly done or undone duties daily. However, if this is done inefficiently it causes more issues worse of it being a falsification of entries. This issue involves a Carer who has been allocated to complete food and fluid intake at the end of every meal time but then the allocator failed to note that this particular Carer has been given another task away from the dining room and the only way for this Carer to complete the task is by asking other Carers one by one, what did this resident eat, how much, what else, how much, what did this resident drink, how much. The staff with this information are often busy elsewhere and they don't like being questioned to provide these details and the questioner whose been allocated to fill this chart don't like bothering colleagues or having to pull the information out of them with a fishing tool or interrogate them. So, in most cases, it leads to some Carers falsifying the information that they fill in. The way forward is the gadget that will be given to every Carer and whoever assists someone to eat should open the mobile gadget and put in the amount consumed immediately.

Recruitment process

I have to add this bit, some care homes insist that all applicants are redirected from the job search website to its own official website where they must fill up several pages of the application form as well as attaching their CV before submitting the application. This is absolutely wrong because the same information contained in cv is being filled all over again into the pages of the application form and it takes a greater amount of time to complete at a stage where they do not even know whether or not they will be selected and it's not as if there is anything special about the particular job or care home being advertised. You tend to lose lots of the best Carers due to this. The best thing is to request just cv and then shortlist after you have had a look at them. Then invite the shortlisted candidates to fill in the forms either online or moment before you interview them.

Stress is man-made

Some residents are supposed to be assisted with personal care [pad change], repositioning or turning while in their bed by two Carers working together in synchronized manner in order to boost the safety of residents and Carers. But due to having too many residents and their respective paperwork to do in a limited time, the Carers, as soon as adrenaline begins to kick in, and time begins to choke upon them, would begin to have one Carer turn/reposition/give personal care alone while another Carer is simultaneously doing the paperwork. It is such a subconscious decision by the two Carers which is prompted by time factor and by having too many tasks to do in a short time. The actions/response of management to send text messages such as the following:

"All staff- nobody should ever reposition or turn alone. If it comes to light that anyone does this you will face instant disciplinary action against you".

Such a response will not investigate the reasons behind this. Especially when the Carers receive messages from the same management asking them to do more [bed baths] which takes far more time than the repositioning/turning/personal care [pad change].

"Hi all if M asks for a shower at 4.30am you shower her you do not say it's too early. No matter what time it is if she asks

for a shower you must do it. Also you need to be doing more bed baths for the main house not just the extension. Thanks "

This sort of message asking already stretched Carers to do more often leads to management having to send the earlier message asking Carers to never reposition or turn alone. Now add the third message that warns Carers against taking the paperwork out of residents' rooms and must do paperwork as they go along.

"All staff at night MUST NOT take the paperwork out of the rooms!!! All folders always follow the resident . If double one can tidy room and one do book. No excuses. Anyone caught bringing paper work out will be disciplined. Legal documents have been scribbled on and now are missing daily notes. Fill them out as you go along pls. Thanks *Thanks***"**

These should give you a clearer picture of what a dilemma the Carers are boxed into. The last text encourages them to do these things alone in a very clear manner and in contradiction of earlier messages. The management will be running around dealing with symptoms of understaffing which causes Carers to subconsciously accept substandard approach to doing too many things at very limited time, but management never actually discusses the staffing issue.

More useful tips

Put a thinking cap on always: The home decided to change the laundry room key which had been broken for a while. There is a specific or unique type of key used in various parts of the home to ensure only permitted individuals to access such rooms, that is a coded lock the one you type in a set of codes to unlock. Very efficient since all staff are informed of the Master code. Now they changed the laundry coded lock and replaced it with a different lock that requires a key to be inserted in order to unlock the door. The problem is that the key is kept in the admin office. So, Carers are expected to collect the key from the admin office each time they need to go into the laundry and return it to the admin office afterwards. The reality is that Carers avoided the laundry room seriously and they keep the laundry room unlocked for many hours. These are such examples of avoidable inefficiencies in practice. A certain colleague and I went to change a resident when we noticed her knickers were wet and need changing, no spare knicker in her drawers means her family had failed to provide enough spare knickers so we needed to go to the laundry basket in laundry room to check for any washed spare in her own laundry basket. My colleague simply went to another resident's room and brought someone else a knicker. I felt bad when I asked why, she responded that we are on the far end of the building, she isn't going to the admin to get the key and then go laundry to check for knickers and then lock laundry and return the key back to the admin office and then bring clean knickers here for us. I understood her point, but we just must go round the building adding up our frustration and fatigue.

Keep master key of out bunch and in one permanent place or use coded locks

Biggest danger related to care home fires is residents locking themselves in their own rooms while they sleep, probably to stop other wandering residents from getting in. The reason for the danger is Carers can only use a master key which is kept in the office but not at a particular point in emergency situations it might take forever to find it, and after that the particular master key will be kept with a bunch of over a dozen other keys. With a coded lock, Carers can get in by typing in the numeric codes only and simply.

Keep plastics [bin bags] out of laundry room

This high temperature laundry room is where the clothes covered in red plastic bags for infection control measure are kept sometimes right next to the boiler tank. This remains a serious fire hazard.

Care home Restructuring

To reduce risks of fire, the laundry room and the kitchen of all care homes should be detached from the rest of the house if possible or located in the farthest corner of the house with two doors separating them from the rest of the house and with no room above them and with a smoke proof ceiling.

Glasses, dentures must be labelled (owner's name/initials engraved on it) by manufacturers

Glasses are prescribed and cannot be shared. Lots of residents' glasses are often not labelled and before you know it, it gets swapped with someone else and there is no way to tell which is which. This is a very serious problem which no one cares about hence it repeats quite often. The question is should unlabelled eyeglasses or dentures be found; whose liability is it to confirm accurate identification of the rightful owner if the resident cannot? It takes a great amount of time asking every staff and resident who a piece of clothing or glasses belong to.

Supplies: there have been days when Carers had to purchase washing up liquid, shower gels etc from their own pocket because when their supplies do not arrive, they suffer for it. If these come from local authorities, then huge pressure should be put on them to cut the bureaucracy and schedule effective series of monthly delivery for residents. If the shower gel comes from the power of attorney, the same sort of pressure should be applied.

Daily notes: updating daily notes takes time, finding the daily notes page inside the large folder on its own scatters the folder and reduces its shelf life and isn't easy, therefore the daily notes should be placed on page one and number one in folder content since it is most used and updated up to four times every 24 hours. This saves time and makes sure your folder lasts long.

Avoid too much repetition; there are some care homes where one information is to be written in 5 different forms.

Duplicate paperwork recording should be banned

I do recognise the need to record what Carers do but I am against the inefficient duplication recording whereby cares are forced to record one information into several forms and folders. In most cases the time required for these duplications is not acknowledged or budgeted by the management. Carers sometimes spend time after their shifts have ended to complete the duplication recordings and if they go home without completing it, they will be asked to come back to work to get it done before going home.

Text messages such as this one, **"All staff Please ensure when a pad change is done that you physically write pc or pad change as well as ticking the appropriate box. Thanks for your support Thanks"**. It required Carers to tick the box in one sheet of table form in one page and write the same information in another page.

A homecare Carer was bitterly complaining to me that they are expected to record what they did for each resident in their respective booklets in their homes (at work) but her problem was that they are also expected to strenuously complete the same information onto their mobile phone application when they get home (at home). The reason why they do it when they get home is because the time needed to do these duplicate sets of recording was unpaid and unaccounted for. I questioned her further and she reasonably said that a 30 minutes call is certainly not sufficient to do everything that they are meant to do for a resident and records these duplicate sets of records.

This creates a bad attitude towards work and it starts all the way from the recruitment stage when Carers are expected to fill in the same information contained in their CV into an application form, you will lose count how many times you have written your name and personal details. Then during each shift in some care homes, you will fill form for each resident with details of the care that you have provided and general welfare of the resident after each interaction or intervention and then you will also write a detailed note of the exact same information that you have just filled into a well detailed rows and columns of the form. Then you do an observation form where you record exactly what you have recorded in the general welfare form and then the food and fluid chart and then record it all over again in the hand over booklet.

This duplication does cause dispute among staff. I had an exchange of words with a nurse one morning after I had almost finished a 12-hours night shift. She said she needed an information regarding which resident opened the bowel during the shift so she could write it in the handover booklet and hand it over to the morning team who will be starting. When I told the nurse which resident had bowel movement, she asked if I documented it in their respective folders to which I replied that I did. She asked which part of the folder where I documented it and I explained that documented it on the part of the resident's folder that asked Carers to tick the box if the resident had a bowel movement and also to indicate whether it was loose bowel or other type according to 'Bristol stool chart'. The nurse demanded that I go back to each resident's room and write it in the summary daily notes if they opened the bowel and the type. I paused and then asked her, that same information you will verbally inform the day team in a minute at hand over, and I can see you just wrote it in the handover booklet now, and I have written the same information in the hourly checks wellbeing form where the same bowel movement question was asked but you still think these weren't enough and I should go room by room to also write it in the summary daily notes probably making it up to two sentences. I am sorry it is almost time to go home so I cannot do that. She was not happy that I disobeyed her orders and stormed out.

Hospitalised residents' paperwork

In my own work, one resident went to hospital in early June 2020 and each day and night a fresh sheet of paper was done for her with the words 'hospitalised' and this went on for the whole month and beyond.

This waste of time is not environmentally friendly, and it happens in every care home. My point is managers often fail to monitor the enormity of paperwork that their Carers are required to do and even when some of the paperwork are absolutely unnecessary, they still continue to do it like robots or zombies just because they fear that not doing so is worse than making the mistake of using their own initiatives.

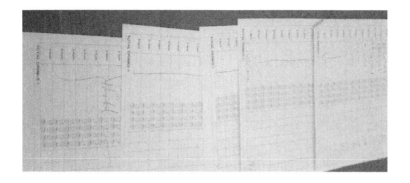

Carers are human beings and must not be degraded like that.

No proper lighting for all that paperwork

This is one big issue for almost every care home that I have been in. The night Carers strain their eyes reading and writing the paperwork, they have no idea how much damage they are doing to their eyes. I once wondered why that was the situation and realised that, there is no light anywhere shining bright enough for reading and writing. Health and safety requirements should include a well-illuminated area of the building where night Carers will be encouraged to read and write it. The problem is that Carers are not given an office, in most cases not given a staffroom and since due to confidentiality issues, they will not be allowed to use the administrative office or the manager's office where certain documents are securely stored. Their only alternative is to write at the dining tables or lounges or conservatory. In these places, the night lighting is not designed for reading or writing. They are little deemed lights to enhance relaxation and deliberately designed to not shine bright.

Paperwork storage

The company could not designate any room for staff to use as staffroom but when the archived paperwork boxes built up to an astounding level, they realised that there is no storage area for it.

Care homes may adopt or convert to cloud storage to reduce the amount of paperwork.

A case for the old-fashioned diary

I sat down with a very unhappy and unsettled gentleman who has dementia and was admitted to our care home on respite. He showed me a diary which his son brought to him the previous day and then he tried to explain his situation to me. The diary helped to make everything make sense to him. He showed me today's date and referred to the previous day when he was admitted and explained to me that he can understand why he was admitted and then said his biggest worry was that his family has not phoned today to give him an update on his wife's health. I can see him reading this diary over and over every time I walked by. I knew immediately that I have learnt something from him and that is the fact that the old-fashioned diary remains to elderly people with dementia what an iPhone (or any other personal digital assistant) is for young adults and teenagers. It is a reminder which helps store that information that the brain cannot store. The fact that it is old fashioned means that it has been known to the elderly people with dementia from childhood, easily recognisable and will take a seriously long time for dementia to spread enough to erase the information stored.

Creating a dementia friendly environment

Many care homes fall short of this and I trace the failure to their neglect of Carers who are on the front line in the battle against dementia. Ask any Carer what dementia residents ask most in your care home and they will tell you. Most residents living with dementia can remember their room number or that they need to go to the toilet but do not remember the directions. So, they will ask any Carer because they can identify the difference between a

Carer and a fellow resident. I will suggest that care homes provide the following.

Location/venue and description; residents should be able to see a signpost indicating the name and location of the care home and show that the property is a care home.

Ease of finding your own way; every corner of the house should be labelled and signposts indicating where it leads to. At the beginning of each corridor, there should be a signpost of the various rooms and facilities such as toilets or lifts or kitchenette or lounge in that corridor.

Comprehensive Clock; clocks that are big enough to be seen, more than one in the lounge & in every room and should indicate time, what next in terms of agenda (e.g. bedtime or activities time or meal times), day/night, day of the week and date. The agenda can be set to promote fluid intake or exercises, good night sleep or even activities and mealtimes. The clock should tell it as well as indicating it since some resident struggle to see.

Lighting and colourings; a resident who can remember his room number for instance room 10 should be further helped if the room's entrance door is painted yellow and different from other rooms in the corridor. And with proper lighting, it should not be difficult to navigate around. These reduce residents with dementia annoying other residents by wandering about and opening their doors. It will not completely stop it, but it will reduce it.

The bedrooms should further be labelled to indicate the light switches, call bell system & its use.

Should have gone to Specsavers

Lack of Effective communication is the biggest setback in the fight against dementia. Residents with dementia would struggle to understand what a Carer is saying when the resident heard the

Carer clearly not to mention when the resident did not hear the Carer. This often leads to the Carer repeating all his or her sentences over and over and talking louder and louder which fast increases the level of stress of the Carer and drains Carer of energy. It eventually leaves the resident feeling lost/isolated because, after a while, Carers, relatives and other residents in the surrounding environment will struggle to have enjoyable interaction especially a chatting section with such a resident and will give up eventually attempting to interact. The problem Carers struggle to understand is why such a resident did not have a hearing aid? The hearing aids help improve hearing hence a very essential need. The most common reason for residents' lack of hearing aid is a loss. To prevent the loss of hearing aid, the hearing aid must have security threads to be used to fasten it to the clothing of the wearer to prevent loss of this expensive miniature item. It may also contain technology or material that should make it glow in the dark.

Ensure handovers are not disrupted

Handover is a very important briefing before the beginning of a shift and very essential for care to remain continuous. The handover session is very important, but a very large number of care homes do not recognise several disruptions and distractions. The first problem is that no time is allocated for all members of the incoming team to have their handover before they start. I will discuss this after. The next problem is that due to the fact that confidential information will be likely to be shared, handover needs to be done in a suitable place but many care homes do not care or do not pay attention and allow handover to be taken in the dining rooms, lounges and other areas where lots of residents are present and can hear the discussion. The next problem is that some residents due to their mental condition may walk into the handover session and distract or disrupt it. In extreme circumstances, I recall this handover where the two nurses were sharing the table with two residents and the three Carers sat in a row of seats behind the four in the same table.

On another day, the handover was done in the administration office, the outgoing day Carers disrupted the handover by walking in every minute to sign out and say goodbye with some chit chats. Their team needs to sign out when times up but that is exactly when the incoming team will be having a handover and the signing out distracts the handover process. Remember proper handover and first thorough safety checks of all residents & environment are key to a successful incident-free shift.

Decorations

Leather upholstery is better than cotton

A new Carer started her first shift, all was going well for her until she sat down in a cotton covered lounge chair not knowing it was soaked in urine. She was very sad we offered her a resident's trouser and a brand-new unused hospital single use underwear to use for the night as we could not allow her to go home. When you see Carers sitting on the arm of a lounge chair or on the side tables, the reason is that they have various times sat-in cotton fabric based non-leather lounge chairs and got their trousers or skirts soaked up in urine. If it were a leather chair, they would notice that it is wet and needs cleaning and sterilising. When foam (cotton covered cushions) get soaked on urine, it cannot be washed. It adds up to give care homes a bad ammonia-like smell after some time or let say, months. In most cases, Carers detach the cushion if it is detachable or the whole chair if the cushion is not detachable and take it outside to the garden, and after some weeks, rain & snow would have fallen on it and it can no longer be returned to the home, you can then see where that fly-tipped rubbish near care homes originate from. Similarly, a resident's mattress should be waterproof material for the same reason explained above. A waterproof polymer material is fine if it is covered over with a cotton bed sheet. Quilts should be waterproof polymer material but must be covered over with cotton quilt covers.

Cover all polymer (tarpaulin) Materials in beds with cotton materials

One resident at this care home where I went to work had a sore knee, which was a bit unusual part of the body for bed sores. It appears that her bed width was small, and she was tall with legs bent because of her shrunken muscles due to her being bed-bound. Anyway, this led to her knee touching the bedside rail either way she turned. The tarpaulin cover of the bedside rails being non-skin friendly gave her a sore knee during the summertime when temperatures rose. The tarpaulin materials being used in bed's mattresses, pillows, bedside rails, heel elevator pillows, etc are all alright except for the fact that the pillowcase and bed sheets are provided to cover pillows and mattresses respectively but the rest of the tarpaulin materials in the bed which makes contact with the bed occupant remain uncovered for reasons that I don't know.

Carpets

Rugs are not for care homes. Rugs smell and absorb urine fast. Use tiles or similar carpet to ease cleaning and drying.

Wastage

Some Care Home staff including seniors and managers are often too careless and/or immature enough to treat care homes furniture and other things with care. They would take a dining chair outside to sit down or spend time outdoors with a resident but then leave the furniture out there till the rain falls and soak it up and then it gets thrown away. Carers must improve on this. Fly-tipping is also a big problem around care home environments and the council has a lot to do to deter people from repeating this situation. Broken furniture and used clothes can be seen scattered around care homes.

Another source of waste is pigeon droppings on garden Furnitures which are kept below trees in the garden. Since no Carer or domestic would clean them, they become waste. If they could all be covered with waterproof or any polymer material, then they may last longer.

Carers' ranking and promotion

The NHS has a way of rewarding long-term relationships with their workers by increasing their band levels as years of service goes by and expected service experience that will be accrued. Their Carers and nurses have different bands such as band 1, band 2 etc. There is usually only one team leader (senior Carer) in every shift which means that the rest of the team members, even those with decades of experience are classified on the same level as a starter on his or her first day of work. This is wrong but because promotion and recognition of length of service are expected to be reflected in the per hour pay rate, companies, therefore, are not interested. The team leader is not a rank. It is an appointed person who has leadership skills and should not be the highest rank that any Carer could attain. A Carer with ten years' experience can be under a team leader with five years of experience but the years of experience should be recognised. If it requires any steps to verify that the Carer has been in an inactive health care job for years, then the verification should be done during set employment. It is nothing but the right thing to do to rank and promote Carers from one level to another. The CQC in collaboration with the NHS and Human Resource Management professor of any UK University should specify the ranking nature or guidelines.

Dealing with relatives and visitors

Management, please stop worshipping relatives

Please stop worshipping relatives. Stop worshipping the ground they walk. The notion that customers are always right does not have to be at the expense of your Carers and does not apply to relatives as they are not customers. They are rather stakeholders alike and have their own responsibility beyond finance. The warning notice should be put up in clear view at entrance to state that any visitor who verbally, physically or in any other means abuse a staff on duty or not or vandalise the property due to being refused entry or delay in allowing entry or any other reason will be prosecuted by relevant authority as the care home would press charges and the person would receive outright ban from visiting the property.

Visitors who themselves need care

An elderly gipsy gentleman visits his son who is our resident almost every day, and during each visit, he would rudely demand food at meal times turning deaf ears to any explanation that residents must all have their own food first and he can get food if there's still any food left. He also demands hot drinks and never says 'please', and he often points his walking stick at Carers when he speaks or complains about his son not being taken to the toilet and assisted with personal care first before every other resident. All the Carers believe without proof that he may have dementia. He can use the toilet; however, he walks slowly while going to the toilet which means that he urinates all over the floor from the corridor to the toilet before he gets to the toilet. The issue is that he is not the care home responsibility and the care home Carers are paid to look after his son but not him but in reality, it appears that the Carers must mop the floor of the toilet and nearby corridor and disinfect the chair he sat on every day that he visits and finally put up with his rude behaviours. This has been a reoccurring issue in every care home because it never gets addressed permanently. When care homes admit an individual, the individual becomes their responsibility. This does not extend to the individual's relative. Managers should discuss with the relatives about it and if the visitor needs care, then they should come up with an arrangement either visit with their own Carers or pay for care while at the premises. Also, certain details should be shared such as the visitor's GP and medical history and existing medical condition. This situation makes Carers feel bad and it may adversely impact the level of compassionate care that they provide.

Dignity and respect are reciprocal

Carers are trained and compelled to treat residents as well as other stakeholders with respect and dignity. But should such treatment not be reciprocated, then it should be taken seriously.

Meeting, training and orientation

Residents and relatives' orientation

There are numerous reasons why residents that have capacity and their families need adequate orientation before being admitted to a care home. This will help create a very clear understanding of both parties' perspectives and expectations. This orientation should highlight the critical points where conflicts emerge as well as the policy and procedure of the company. This orientation must be compulsory attendance. Issues raised in this memoir could help in some ways.

Use simple words in online training

Total disregard of the fact that most Carers who will be using this learning platform are not well educated below college in the UK. The use of words such as.

'inadvertently' a word that can easily be substituted with popular and easily understood words.

Another related issue is the unnecessary sophistication of Carers' online training. Below is a question in one of my training and it shows extremely and unnecessary sophistication and complexity. "Question 5: How do Acetylcholinesterase Inhibitors work to treat Alzheimer's?

A. Lowering the levels of Acetylcholine in the brain

B. Preventing Acetylcholinesterase from breaking down acetylcholine in the brain

C. Blocking the activity of the neurotransmitter glutamate

D. Activating glutamate in the brain"

From this question, one may assume that I was training to be a biochemist at undergraduate or postgraduate level. The question itself indicates that a poor Carer like me has a strong interest in Alzheimer related research, pharmacology or Biochemistry. How will my knowledge of 'Acetylcholinesterase' help me in my job of caring for someone with dementia? How long after this training will I even remember this word, 'Acetylcholinesterase'? This unnecessary sophistication extends the training time, and this is an unpaid time, my own time to spend with my family while at home.

One cloud database for all training

A Carer has a long list of training to do and renew annually. The problem is that Carers being on low income jobs, do often have more than one job. This means that each of their employers will want them to do these training sessions. Since the employer is paying, they will refuse to issue each certificate copy of the training to their Carers. There is also the issue of Carers keeping their second jobs secret. These reasons mean that a Carer will have to do the same training repeatedly. Considering that they often attend or do online training in their spare time off work or attend training sessions while at work thereby putting burden on their teammates. It also means that there is a huge waste of time and effort and money in these training sessions. The local safeguarding or CQC should arrange a similar training database just like the DBS update service where all Carers' training will be stored, updated by any accredited training provider and employers can easily download certificates or arrange for their Carers to attend only trainings that are relevant to them.

Give Carers' their training certificates

Copies of all training certificates which Carers undertook while at any employment must be issued to them immediately such training is completed. Care Homes must stop withholding Carers ' training certificates as a ransom or any other purpose as it belongs to the Carer. It should be unlawful to deny Carers access to copy documents bearing the Carer's name such as certificates.

Medical cream directions of use and body map
This is a very overlooked one, Carers often do not know exactly where creams are meant to be applied. This information which should be written on the cream container in a body map format is rather kept confidential in the administration office of most care homes. considering that a temporary Carer would not know where this information is stored and would not be bothered to search for it before applying cream on a resident, this information is best kept on the medication itself rather than the normal note on creams which states, "apply to affected areas", the focus areas should be stated clearly on the medical cream container.

Body lotion training
In December of 2019, I saw my name on the board to attend a certain training course titled 'Cavillon training'. To understand my situation, I take two buses to work. To cut long story short, the Cavillon-cream is a cream brand that helps keep skin healthy and this training was aimed at teaching Carers how to apply the cream. But the honest question was why it cannot be done during work hours. Show the Carers on duty and so on. The training is good, but the schedule was terribly wrong. It was very insensitive mandating Carers to not spend their time-off with their families and attend a training that could simply be achieved in an easier alternative.

Lesbian, gay, bisexual and trans (LGBT) residents
I have noticed that the number LGBT residents living in care homes is quite larger than the system acknowledged. Their situation is far more difficult because they are more likely to be discriminated against by their fellow residents and some staff.

Having grown up in an era where the society discriminated, pathologized and maltreated LGBT people, they are less likely to identify themselves as LGBT now than younger people. They are likely to still hide their sexuality from fellow residents and their care homes. If they do not come out, there is risk of such people facing alone such specific challenges that follows not being open, not feeling free, fear of being abandoned by relatives as well as other negative perceptions. They will be too reserved to use certain services or seek help. This will adversely affect the care home's ability to meet their long-term needs. But then even if they do come out, none of the Carers have received any LGBT specific training that is solely based on understanding and not being judgemental. The equality and diversity training which Carers receive is too vague for this. Care homes try to appear LGBT friendly by having LGBT material clearly showing or using images that represent people from the LGBT community but without training the staff, they will not be aware and sensitive and avoid being judgemental. Care homes only began awareness of this seriously important issue in late 2017 and early 2018 but as of 2020, this awareness dried up. The awareness which was just a memo posted on the general notice board that our care home is LGBT friendly appears to be the end of the matter and nothing else has been done. No staff training and no extra box has been created in all sexuality forms used for residents to indicate sexuality or any form of encouragement for LGBT residents to feel free to come out and stay out.

Sexual Harassment should be a training module
I must point out that I was never accused of harassing anyone sexually, but I have seen it happen at various times in care homes where I worked. In the care home environment, colleagues work together, stress up together, take the piss & do the job absorbing

the ups and downs that come with it together and giving each other a shoulder to lean on. Colleagues find themselves spending 12 hours on a stretch together in one building day by day or night by night. The issue of flirting with each other, playing with each other including physical contacts or discussing erotic/Sexual subjects or having a good laugh is extremely rampant as the stressful nature of the job leads Carers to higher cigarette smoking, high caffeine level from drinking coffee or adrenaline level of the body demands letting off some steam and this becomes dangerous due to the fact that almost all of the Carers do not know exactly the boundaries in terms of what actions by law is regarded as Sexual Harassment. A female Carer sees a male Carer sitting down and would sit on his lap without permission or hug a male Carer or even jump on him, female Carers hugging male residents appear to be normalised and no one minds, male Carers would playfully touch a girl's hair or put arms around her shoulder. One moment there may be flirting and so on then the next minute the frustration of the job kicks in leading up to disagreement and mild fall out and subsequent Sexual harassment allegations. The issue is that when they are all having a laugh, it seems alright but as soon as a misunderstanding which has nothing to do with Sexual Harassment arose, then one of the parties who felt hurt would use Sexual Harassment allegations to get back at the other party and when those various playful moments are narrated in presence of management and under a Sexual Harassment context, it is very easy to put the other party in an extremely vulnerable position despite the fact that these flirting may have been totally mutually desired when it occurred. In other times, the playing and flirting gets misinterpreted as an indication of attractiveness which if one of the parties makes a further move, a very bad reject will bring catastrophic awkwardness to the team going forward and the impact of a subsequent fall out will be very devastating to the team.

Moving and Handling training for residents

If you leave every knowledge of a car to the mechanics and none to drivers, the rate of accidents will multiply. But then why leave every knowledge of safe moving and handling manoeuvre to only the Carers and none to residents? "Pull me up or find me someone who will". This quote for instance causes more misunderstandings and problems in the daily work of every Carer. It is a spoken request to be pulled up, made by a resident who feels he or she cannot on his or her own strength and effort stand up. Why won't a Carer simply pull a resident up?

Why would a resident expect to be pulled up by a Carer in such a situation as described above? The answers to these questions come from professional moving and handling of individuals training which every Carer (but not residents) must undergo in order to safely do his or her job without causing injuries to him or herself or to the resident. This training is supposed to dwell on this issue or scenario as detailed and clear as possible. Carers should at the end of the training understand that pulling an elderly resident by the arm risks dislocating the resident's arm from the shoulder and it is therefore illegal as well as being an abuse of a resident. There are many other ways that are used in the past to pull people up but are banned and condemned today because such manoeuvres risk causing injury to the Carer. The common sense involved in this situation is that large scale research has been conducted and various equipment designed to help pull up anyone living in the care home should the person not be able to 'get self-up'. On the other hand, imagine a Carer pulling every resident up any resident who requests to be pulled up, the manager of the care home would have regular work injury related diagnosis, lawsuits and compensation to pay out since Carers would be acquiring lots of injuries while working. According to the training, only paramedics or fire service personnel in emergency situations can pull people up while trying to save them. But why is the equipment which is readily available not being used? The reason is, Carers have a great deal of equipment to use to pull or lift residents up if the need arises. The palaver is that the equipment is reserved for residents who genuinely need it (rather than conveniently or due to laziness) following a duly conducted assessment by a qualified senior member of staff. The biggest misunderstanding is that residents do not know why Carers just will not pull them when asked and almost all of them see it as Carer being mean and refusing to help them no matter how the Carer tries to explain. This problem is escalated when badly or untrained Carers pull residents up when asked therefore when other well-trained Carers refuse to do it, the resident is very likely to take it personal and unlikely to understand whatever explanation the trained Carer may give. Residents sometimes say things like, "my son pulls me up with just a hand" or they would rudely ask the Carer to leave their room to go and call someone else since the resident believes that the Carer was just being mean. Some residents do threaten to report the Carer for refusing to pull him or her up. Carers take threats extremely seriously and any resident using threat risks losing compassion from the Carer being threatened.

These are very real sources of grievances and occur on a very regular basis every day. Earlier I mentioned giving new residents and relatives orientation and induction so that these issues will be clearly explained. Moving and handling of people is totally deemed to be training for Carers but take a closer look at this, human beings learn to stand, then walk, but then at old age when they need to learn and to adapt to the changes and challenges of their body's mobility and movement, another individual will receive the training and induction and orientation needed while the person who owns the body is completely left out. A manager or senior may observe the resident and update the resident's care plan and that is it. No orientation on what to expect from the Carers and what is expected of the resident for sustainable personal moving and handling until the next assessment. Health and safety executives have categorised responsibilities according to the Carers', employers' and clients' responsibilities. This is one of the most versatile and most important analyses and frameworks that remains useful in ensuring the health and safety of all. The problem is that the employers and the employees are trained and given adequate induction, but the clients are often not. They are not given simpler induction sessions when admitted into the home. Residents who have the capacity do not even know what to do in events of fire or emergencies or during hoisting manoeuvres etc Residents should take part in moving and handling training because they are involved in the manoeuvre.

Why Night care staff rarely attend day meetings

Let us say there is a general meeting today at 2 pm, all staff must attend. For night staff, it's Either they have finished a shift earlier in the morning and likely will be asleep in bed in the afternoon or they have a shift tonight so need to get some sleep before commencing to ensure they stay up all night. Either way, they or most of them cannot attend this afternoon meeting.

Since they are fewer than day staff, there must be a way of achieving the desired objective - this needed discussion with the management. The meeting for day staff can hold once but the manager should hold meetings with night staff just as they arrive for their shift maybe 30 minutes earlier than the start of shift and repeat the same meeting for another set of night staff on the following night. This is also the way to do fire drills in order to ensure all staff take part and know what to do in times of fire.

General advice

The 'weightlifting belt' myth

It is very unfortunate that the most important thing that isn't taught or discussed during 'moving and handling of people' training is Carer's belt that is worn to basically hold the trouser firmly in place as well as the myth surrounding the weightlifting belt also known as the abdominal belt which many believe to help reduce work-related back injury. Does the way a Carer puts on his or her waist trouser belt increases or reduces the risk of lower back injury? What should a Carer avoid?

Does the 'weightlifter belt' also known as 'abdominal belt' help reduce or prevent the risk of work back injury? The UK health and Safety executive and the CQC must conduct medical research to find out if these should be encouraged or discouraged in terms of its use as personal protective equipment (PPE). I have never used or discussed with anyone who has so I must remain in the one I know well which the everyday belt is used solely to hold my trousers in place. I have observed that I get more back injury when I wear a very non-flexible leather belt and especially if I wear it very low beneath my waist. However, if I wear a little stretchy or elastic sort of belt above my waist, I am usually alright, and it will hold my trouser in an excellent position. Personally, I would recommend a stretchy/elastic belt for one purpose of holding your trouser in an excellent position which should be right up above the waist to give your legs and its associated muscles the unhindered flexibility it needs. I do not fasten it tight but just enough to stop it falling from the exact position where I want it to be. What I actually did, I took out the elastic from my old underwear that had served its purpose, cut a hole each side of my new black chinos I bought for work and pushed the elastic through it and used a thread to hold each of the holes and the elastic together. Then I realised that I did not need the belt anymore. The elastic gave me excellent flexibility.

Burglary
Stealing staff handbags while in staff rooms
Targeting control drugs and residents' wedding rings and other jewellery.
This book certainly would not be possibly written had I complied and kept my phone in the staff room. I had to write many things down right after it had happened and safely use the phone and that was the only way to ensure that I did not forget.

Armed Robbery
Many armed robbers attack Carers usually armed with knife or other weapons and their main target is usually the control drugs. Once the robber(s) get into the building, they would threaten the Carers with weapon demanding that they hand over the control drugs locker keys and point them to where it is. The Carers must be brave and risk injuries to themselves or just let the robber(s) have their way which means carting away with the control drugs. Carers have never received training or guidance on how to react or respond during such incident. They do not have a clue what not to do or what best to do. There should be a security training for such incident.

After party diarrhoea
It is a recurring incident that four out of five care home partying results in some residents' diarrhoea the morning after. Halloween, Christmas, Easter, Valentine's Day, birthdays etc.
While waiting for guests' arrival, food is exposed or not stored in the refrigerator during this wait. Hot food will not be temperature probed to ensure it is not below the minimal serving

temperature or out of the danger zones. Relatives bring in food which is not verified to be safe before being consumed by residents and the food given to residents are often not reheated. Foods are collected in buffet form. No one has ever attempted to stop this recurrent issue.

Wall Sockets

The wall sockets and/or call bell sockets have this tendency of being broken regularly. It is caused by hospital beds knocking it off when it is being raised to enable staff to provide personal care to the resident on the bed. This can be solved simply by putting a permanent restraint such as a guiding metal or wooden rail to stop the bed from ever getting any closer to the wall in the first place. Alternatively, it can be prevented by fixing the sockets to the wall at a height beyond or beneath the reach of the bed's highest or lowest reachable level.

It is very unfortunate that in some care homes, they threaten or/and in some cases deduct the cost of fixing or replacing a smashed socket from staff wage if a staff forgot to shift the bed away from the wall before lifting the bed up with the wired controller. This callous action does not solve the problem because one day an agency Carer who doesn't know about the danger or risk will just press the button on the wired controller to lift the bed and the socket will certainly get smashed yet again. It can also lead to Carers avoiding the bedroom if they can help it. Not because they dislike the resident, rather no one wants to get their peanut income reduced because of a slight mistake. This will overtime lead to neglect of the resident.

Nail wardrobes to wall

Please nail all wardrobes to the walls to prevent it from falling and hurting any resident or Carer.

Secure fire extinguishers

Due to several incidents involving new unhappy (Usually male) residents, who are not yet ready to accept the situation and be living in a care home, a new review of fire extinguishers in location should be carried out to ensure they are never used as a weapon in times.

Big Wheelchair Tyres

Wheelchair with big radius tyres with its teethed threads is extremely risky for some nursing residents who are not naturally fully aware of their surroundings. Their fingers or skin are too close to the hot fast-moving threads of the moving tyre. They often unknowingly put their fingers rubbing against the moving tyre and some inexperienced Carers might not know about this hazard and in a few seconds later, be looking for where a pool of blood is trailing behind gushing from and see it is from the resident's fingers. Fingers do get trapped in the wheelchair wheel/spoke too.

Avoid locking Doors to keep off wanderers

The issue of wandering residents disturbing other residents during the night by opening their doors thereby waking up the occupant of the room is a very regular occurrence. The response in some cases is that residents lock their doors from the inside and the only way Carers could come in is with the spare/master key. If there is a fire, would Carers remember to tell the fire service personnel that by the way, the key to room 30 is in the office but what if the office is already in flames?

Elevators standard room/space

Elevators in care homes must have a certain standard that they must meet in terms of space to at least have room for a wheelchair maximum size plus Carer who is pushing it. I have just watched a 5-month pregnant colleague squeeze out of the lift. Terrible!

The lift was at this one care home too small for a stand aid and a lady upstairs needed a stand aid to help her stand up. After various Carers had ignored the problem and continued to drag-Lift this lady, I raised this issue with the manager and she promised to get smaller equipment from Red Cross lease/lend or from a sister care home under the same company group. But her promise was never fulfilled for almost a year till the resident passed away. The funny part is that she ensured that all moving, and handling training is up to date for all Carers so that when the CQC visit, they will be satisfied.

In another care home, there isn't any lift and when one of the upstairs equipment is broken then Carers must carry the equipment upstairs and downstairs until the broken one is fixed and you will expect it will be fixed immediately, wrong it took many months.

Side tables are hazards

Most bed falls result in injuries as one would expect. But of all, one injury that I have seen time and time again is residents rolling out of bed and hitting the head on side tables. Some of which are solid oak wood items of furniture. The crash mat can protect residents from hitting hard on the horizontal floor but cannot protect residents from vertical side tables kept next to the bed.

Stop the distrust

I asked my colleague since every day we fill up these lounge water jugs and they're never used up to half by the time we take them back to washing, what if we stop wasting the squash and fill each of the jugs half way rather than full? She replied, your suggestion is good, but they would suspect we did not change them from last night and suspect we did not wash the jugs, but we simply replaced the covers. On another instance, I asked a colleague, the resident has worn this shirt and cardigan just today, putting it in the washing basket for washing is bad for the fabric, the two items of clothing are clean and smell fresh still. The response I got was, your suggestion is good but since we cannot put them back into her wardrobe mean we have to put them back on her tomorrow morning, the problem is they may insinuate we didn't wash her since she is still having previous day clothes on. On another instance night, Carers switch lights in lounges off during the night to save energy but this had to stop when it was reported that they may have switched the lights off to give themselves a cosy sleep while they sat in the lounge waiting for call bells to go off and to respond. The distrust makes a huge impact on decision making of care staff and this impact leads to wastage.

Fire exit doors are serious escape hazards

The higher the number of fire exit doors without any call bell trigger connection to the central system, the greater the risk of residents absconding from the building unnoticed. A large proportion of escape prevention is usually focused on the front door entrance and this door will have a good locking system, but the most vulnerable escape means remains the fire exit doors. Most fire exit doors have clearly written simplified directions on how to open the door for the purpose of easy escape during a fire emergency.

Resident's escape is very dangerous since a resident wandering in the streets could be hit by a hit & run driver. The reality is that no amount of periodic routine checks or observations can prevent any determined resident from leaving the building through one of these fire exits and not to mention that Carers have other residents to look after. Carers will be likely to expect such a resident to attempt any escape by first coming downstairs and leave through one of the downstairs fire exit doors. This creates a blind spot which is the upstairs fire exit door with a metal staircase which usually leads to the backyard of the property.

It should be an essential criterion for licensing of new care homes for every home to have all fire exit doors or windows connected to the central call bell system in order to alert Carers as soon as one is opened. A stitch in time saves nine. In event of residents escaping, please go easy on the Carers and avoid sweating (questioning them as if you are interrogating them or threatening to do this or that or to take the incident forward) them over it since a basic alarm system connection to the central call bell system could have prevented the escape from happening in the first place. It is also worth noting that on a single occasion, a resident renowned for several attempted escapes couldn't be found, the police had to send a helicopter to hover around the area and at the end he was found hiding in his wardrobe.

Successful resident escape

On this 8pm to 8am night shift, a resident was very unsettled and kept looking for a door to leave the building from 9pm. There were only two of us Carers looking after over 20 residents. We also had to clean and mop the kitchen, three lounges, dining, toilets and the laundry. So, we certainly have a lot to do and there is no way we could have kept one to one eye on him all night.

We tried to keep an eye on him and twice he opened the fire exit in the lounge and left the building as each of us were assisting other residents into their respective beds and as soon as we returned we looked for him only to realise that he had opened the fire exit and closed it properly to prevent detection and we brought him back just as he was attempting to climb the wooden fence. The second time he tried the same thing again, he got injured by the fence and we convinced him to go upstairs with us to his bedroom for treatment. While there, we stopped the bleeding with a plaster. We also made him another drink and offered snacks and hoped he stayed in his bed as we had to attend to other residents.

Less than an hour later I saw him walking down the stairs, he saw me and walked backwards in a sort of creepy way, so I followed him discreetly and he watched him go into his bedroom. The time was exactly half past midnight. At one o'clock, the daughter phoned the landline and when we answered she asked why she received calls from a stranger that her dad was at their house. She was very angry and threatened that she 'is taking it further' and said lots of other things to which she later apologised. Her dad was soon brought back to the care home by a neighbour who lives about a few doors away. Urgent check revealed that he had opened an upstairs fire exit door which had a hammer and instruction, made his way to the backyard of the building and either climbed over the brick fence or walked through a broken-down wooden part of the fence. The fire exit door had on it a hammer and clear and precise instructions on how to open it in an emergency.

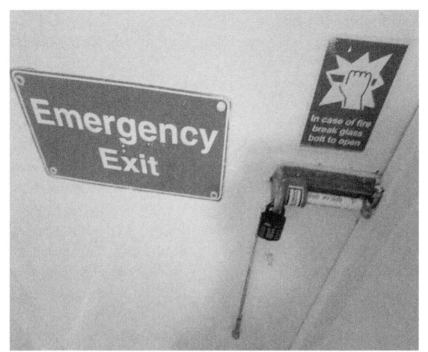

The care home building was not a prison and was not designed to prevent people escaping from it. The man did not have any deprivation of liberty safeguards (DOLs) which means that we had no right to forcefully prevent his escape. In fact, the management only made an application for his DOLs after this incident had occurred using this incident as proof that he needs DOLs. The most heart breaking and horrifying part of it was the blame and threat by his daughter to take it further clearly implying to take whatever actions against us Carers as well as the care home.

Night shifts and breaks

Imagine the fact that care homes put two Carers only to work on a twelve hours night shift looking after over twenty residents or three Carers to look after over 40 residents and at the end, an hour out of their twelve hours will be deducted from their total hours for break by payroll despite them not taking any break during their shift. They never take any breaks for a reason. As a matter of fact, if each of them took their breaks, then it means that for two hours, there will be only one Carer on the shift where two Carers are working while there will only be two Carers for three hours where three Carers are working. The problem is that so many residents are on hourly and bi-hourly turns/tilt to prevent pressure sore and these turns/tilt rounds require at least two Carers working together to do safely. But Carers dare not write in the resident's folder that the turn/tilt was not done because one Carer was on break. This shortage of staff for that two hours is completely normal and undocumented and consequences unassessed or unknown. There are consequences such as Carers falsifying to have done the turn when they didn't or to have done the turn working with another Carer as it should be done whereas the turn was done by only one Carer which raises extreme risk of manual handling injury. The other consequence is that the lone Carer can only be at one place at any time during the two hours so therefore if something is going wrong elsewhere, or another resident needs help, no one else will respond. These consequences were highlighted at a particular care home where a Carer who was officially warned against dozing off requested that her officially untaken hour-long break time shall henceforth be taken, and she will time it minute by minute. Her decision to take her break led directly to the point where other Carers wanted their breaks too when on night shift and suddenly it became clear that staff shortage within the staff break time required fixing.

Exhaustion/Fatigue is a good enough reason

Carers are treated with very serious scepticism when they ring sick. The reason behind this is that they are not allowed to take time off when they have fatigue. Night staff often must go to work whether they have had a very tiresome day. Fatigue affects Carers' response time. Rather than an NHS falls prevention training for all staff, simply recognise that late or slow response to buzzer/call bells is due to exhaustion and recognise that the job requires a great deal of physical activity. Standing on the feet walking, bending, and pulling or pushing for over 2 hours nonstop. Carers now get Fitbit to monitor distances they walk, and it is lots of miles. Since football coaches leave players, they pay hundreds of thousands per week sitting on side-lines during games, why must Carers tell lies of diarrhoea to be allowed off when the core reason is exhaustion? I have spoken to a colleague who has a college student husband/partner and she told me she finishes work and starts childcare for her daughter and rarely sleeps before it's time to start working again and at times she does get seriously exhausted and that is the plain innocent truth. She told me these while we were working together and now, she was over halfway through another pregnancy.

In some care homes, Carers when they phone in sick, they are forced to turn up for meetings with the manager as a way of eradicating 'falsely calling in sick'. Carers must turn up to work despite being or claiming to be sick and then go back home supposedly after proving to the manager with symptoms in obvious fashion.

Furthermore, a memo is usually circulated in several care homes in the beginning of December threatening Carers against calling in sick in the entire month in general and in bank holidays of the month.

In most care homes, Carers do not get paid 'sick pay' for missing a shift or two due to illness. Most Carers are threatened that should they phone-in sick, they will be investigated by the management to verify their claim. If they phone-in sick up to a certain amount of times they will be issued with a warning in the form of threats of disciplinary action in obvious indication that the management believes that the Carer claims of being sick were false.

In physics, it is called error due to parallax

Accept that there should be room for error. I got home in the morning from a night shift and went to the bathroom to have a shave and a shower. While shaving I gave my chin a big cut and realised that my eyes may be open, but I am not awake. I had another similar occurrence when trying to get an ATM card from my phone wallet after a night shift, I dropped my phone but luckily the screen didn't crack but I once again understood that my eyes were open but I wasn't awake. A colleague told me that she barely had 3 hours sleep before her alarm woke her up to get ready for another night shift and she walked straight to the bathroom to shower without realising that she was not wearing any clothes at all and she did walk past her son's bedroom.

Carers' management should recognise this and allow room for error. Certain mistakes should not be seriously punished as if they were deliberate or as a result of a Carer's carelessness.

Sleeping while on a waking night duty

This is a very controversial issue. I would like to make it clear that my point here remains that perpetually sleeping while on duty is gross negligence however, feeling too tired or too sleepy on one night or falling asleep should not be any reason for disciplinary action. One would deem sleeping on duty to be gross negligence but the fact that the care industry needs more workers and in a critical shortage of workforce shows that the industry cannot pick and choose. Before you read this part, I would like you to first read the part above which I titled, 'Exhaustion/Fatigue is a good enough reason to phone in sick'. It is very important to treat Carers who sleep while on duty the same way we treat Carers who come to work despite being sick with non-contagious medical conditions. We try to encourage them and accommodate them and give them choices of either going home (or calling them an ambulance to take the Carer to the hospital) or they will be allowed to take a break and go to the staff room to rest and continue afterwards if that's what the staff prefer. We show appreciation for the resilience to continue to work despite the illness and not letting the team down. The same treatment should be given to staff who are found to be asleep while on a night shift. I can assure you that it is far better to treat the body's severe urge to sleep by obliging and napping for 20 minutes than to spend the entire night fighting with the body and nature's call. I hate to hear that a manager suspended a night Carer following a report by a fellow night Carer that the suspended staff was found asleep in the chair during the night shift. This action is totally unacceptable. There is no human being who has not out of utter exhaustion collapsed and collapsing should not be punished. There is no night Carer who has never ever had a night that they struggled to stay awake. If you strictly must suspend any Carer who falls asleep, you will in no time suspend your entire night team. You must make it clear that sleeping on duty is not acceptable, but you must be careful with your punishment for sleeping on duty. Encourage your night seniors to send any Carer found sleeping to go on his or her break.

Feeling sleepy on a night shift should be absolutely recognised as a possibility rather than an unspeakable and despicable situation as currently is. The right measures should be adopted to encourage any staff who feels sleepy to step forward and inform the rest of the team which should be required to help or show solidarity with the staff involved to either take his or her break and sleep it out for an hour and then return back to work feeling very awake or to call a taxi and go home. However, perpetually sleeping on far too many times should prompt the management to not discipline the staff but offer a choice of switching on to the day shift or reducing the number of nights in a week or in a row for the staff to see if it will help the staff to solve the problem.

Flexible rota

Night Carers can do without being stuck in the traffic the morning after. The problem is that most of them need to be home, look after children, get some sleep and return to work in the night. Failing to get enough sleep before returning to work in the evening leads to feeling tired and sleepy while on a night shift. Besides, there is a serious risk of a car crash for those who drive.

Choose popular crisps

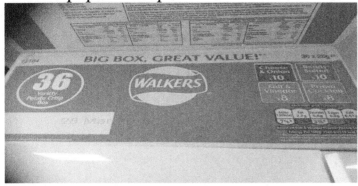

In our care home, the management orders the above box of crisps each time and the x10 cheese and onion, ready salted will be picked by residents leaving behind almost all the salt & vinegar and the prawn cocktail. This important information never gets to the manufacturer and they keep producing the unwanted crisps in large quantities and the problem keeps going round and round. Could somebody please deliver this message to Walkers crisps.

Hard crunchy biscuits

Residents either have weak teeth or wear dentures mostly so please buy very soft biscuits and avoid hard ones such as ginger biscuits.

10 Creams in one resident room and none in another

I walked into a resident's room to assist with personal care (washing and dressing up) and didn't find any 'dry skin' body lotion such as Diprobase cream to put on him but then when I went to his neighbour, I found up to ten such creams and the resident declined to have the cream put on her and it was my responsibility to respect her decision. Now since each of these creams bear her name, they are deemed to be prescribed therefore I will not be permitted to take one off her and give to someone else knowing full well that despite my alerting the person in charge of the shift to arrange a cream for the resident who hasn't got but needs one, it will take a few weeks to get the delivery considering the bureaucracy. But we are talking about something as little as a moisturising body cream, not some blood thinning tablets. The date of recording of this issue is 12th September and I found unopened creams dated 20th of every month as far back as January same year.

Provide wet wipes for cleaning of residents' body
It is very difficult and with very huge friction to clean residents who is incontinent of faeces with tissue paper. Wet wipes are a lot better than tissue papers. The problem is that care homes often fail to provide wet wipes and often fail to provide the required quantity monthly. Some care homes do not provide wet wipes but tell Carers to soak red flannels in water and use it. The issues with using red flannels for this purpose is that the washing machine hardly ever washes the faecal stains off thoroughly even when sluice washed twice thereby presenting a clear risk of infection since the red flannels are shared by all residents. Some Carers do not often stick to red flannels and as a matter of fact use other coloured flannels which are meant for cleaning rest of body of residents to clean the bottom or the other way round whereby some Carers use red flannels to clean resident's face and rest of body contrary to the manager's advice. The best thing is simply to provide toilet-flushable wet wipes or other disposable wet wipes that can be recycled. According to the Independent online news on October 2017, "doctors are warning that wiping alone could leave faeces behind while excessive use could cause health problems such as anal fissures and urinary tract infections". The Independent also reported that Rose George, author of The Big Necessity: The Unmentionable World of

Human Waste and Why It Matters, confirmed that, "Toilet paper moves s***, but it doesn't remove it."

Safeguarding vulnerable adults

Safeguarding should not be safeguarding residents only

Safeguarding' is like a multi-way traffic highway being treated as one-way traffic highway and every now and then two vehicles will collide head-on and you think maybe now the highway will be treated as a two-way traffic highway but still to your greatest surprise, everyone will cast their blames on the symptoms and carry on as usual.

Safeguarding Training

Since being in the industry I have been made to undergo this training annually and this time, I took it out on the trainer for repeating the same training again and again and again without any impact. So, what is wrong with the Safeguarding of vulnerable adults SOVA Training? This is my own version of 'teacher don't teach me nonsense'. To the point, the training is extremely biased in favour of who is perceived as vulnerable adults. The trainer began the training showing us several newspapers and BBC panorama and so on of residents who were abused by their Carers in care homes but paid a very little lip service to the abuse of Carers who are also vulnerable themselves at times at the hand of residents. The trainer used only one slide of the PowerPoint to say all human beings are entitled to a life free of abuse but failed to go any deeper than saying those words and quickly moved to the final slide. I remember an advert I watched on Facebook about a man shouting and pushing his wife in a park and in a minute over 5 individuals were questioning him how dare you to abuse your wife? The same couple swapped places and this time the lady was shouting and pushing her man at the same park and spot for a long time, but no one questioned her. This advert then wrote that in up to 40% of domestic abuse, men were the victim. Residents, as well as children, are classified as vulnerable. Safeguarding training is not just for Carers, teachers also have training for safeguarding vulnerable children training. But does any trainer ever mention that in 2015 two teachers (Ann Maguire who taught Spanish lessons at Corpus Christi Catholic College in Leeds, England and Mr Uzomah, who taught Maths at Dixons Kings Academy in Bradford) were stabbed by their students and one of them died? Carers are abused daily and it often goes unreported. The problem with safeguarding is a poor discussion of those critical issues in care. I questioned the trainer with several scenarios and demanded her response. Only then did she realise how ill-prepared she was and all she said was that Carers should expect to be abused and almost said just like policemen have a thing they call collateral damage. She made mention of her sister who comes home with bruised arms and scratches from working in a nursing home. But I did not know what else to say as she has just contradicted what was in that slide that every individual is entitled to a life free of abuse. Abuse of Carers is not normal so should not be considered to be and the starting point should be to train Carers and encourage them to take it seriously and on how to protect themselves while at the same time protecting their residents from all forms of abuse.

Take this from me to you, abuse in care sometimes is simply the hate that hate produced, the bias that bias produced, neglect that neglect produced, wicked that wicked produced. If everyone acts right, employers truly adopt best practice human resource management, the government properly funds the system, then this could be turned into the love that loves produced and care that care produced. An Igbo proverb says, may the rivers never dry and the fish did not die. You must look after the residents as well as their Carers if you are to succeed in eradicating abuse to a significant extent.

Incomplete definition of 'An adult at risk of harm'

According to definition of an online training centre called 'log on to care eLearning' created by The Grey Matter Group whose mission is improving lives through learning and used by most local councils and charities in England, "an adult at risk of harm is defined as someone who has needs for care and support, and is experiencing, or at risk of, abuse or neglect and is unable to protect themselves". While this definition is correct for care home elderly residents, it failed totally to consider that their Carers may not have needs for care in the same way as residents but they should be considered as people who need care and are also sometimes vulnerable, may be experiencing, or at risk of, abuse or neglect and are unable to protect themselves from their residents, management and third party (relatives). This is a good instance of a one-sided and biased perspective of abuse which is not sustainable. This training listed modern slavery as a type of abuse and I remember vividly, in 2016, I advised 2 Bulgarian fresh immigrant Carers to phone the police when they told us they work for a recruitment agency that provided their overcrowded accommodation, work and transportation from Bulgaria to the UK but continue to take up to 90% of their monthly income. They can speak very little English so without this recruitment agency they will struggle to get another job or accommodation in the UK. I told them it is human trafficking. These Carers are at risk of harm, but the above definition did not take them into consideration.

Safeguarding care home pets

Safeguarding vulnerable adults has been so prioritised that everything else could be neglected. There are very high incidents of care home animals (pets) in care homes dying out of neglect.

It is very sad. I have seen far too many in different care homes. A situation where the fish tank filter takes ages to be replaced and the fish died due to the polluted water not to mention the stench. The bird cages rarely get cleaned and the birds never get visited by a veterinary expert. CQC inspectors do not seem to consider it as part of their job. The RSPCA should do something about this by creating an agreement with the CQC. There should be a mandatory reporting of such incidents to the RSPCA by the care home as part of its duty of care in order to monitor the health and safety of animals in care homes. If the Carers are well overworked and their shifts understaffed, any pets are less likely to be looked after by the same struggling Carers because their priorities remain residents first. On the other hand, if the management does not have a well-planned routine to have professional veterinary care provided to the pets, then the pets will not survive and that is neglect and animal cruelty. Pets need care. Pets are not mandatory for care homes to have. If it cannot be looked after, then it should be unlawful to keep them. CQC should check the welfare of all care homes pets and question how many died in preceding years and when they were last seen by veterinary professionals.

The Blame-the-Carer factor

I find it wrong that residents are completely free of any or all responsibilities and are never accorded any blame. In various cases, someone just must be blamed. Management, relatives and social workers must stop blaming the Carers or finding unfounded faults with the manner which Carers safely handle or report serious incidents and avoid harm from happening to either them or the resident. Let us look at few real-life situations.

1. A Carer once narrated her experience to me; how she was grabbed by her resident who began to take off his belt, the Carer

asked him, why are you taking off your belt and he replied, you need to be whipped. According to the Carer, she held both hands and made him sit down in a chair behind him and quickly detached herself from him. She was blamed for doing so and she said she got furious and said to her manager, "there's no way I'm getting whipped for £7.20 an hour" which was a minimum wage at the time the incident occurred. Not long after, the resident was moved to more secure facility on Christmas day after another incident when he began to destroy the properties of the care home including smashing the TV etc, the director and manager where phoned to come and help and the resident went after them on their arrival that they ran to the office, locked themselves in and told Carers to phone police quickly. The Carers having to phone the director and manager to come in and witness the situation shows a lack of confidence to deal with the situation by phoning the police probably for fear of being blamed.

2. An incident involving a self-neglecting resident who was being shaved by a Carer was read by the social worker who was fuming that the Carer should not have used the word 'dangerous' and summoned the Carer for some sort of telling off/interrogation. According to the Carer, the social worker said to him that the word 'dangerous' is to be used if the resident was chasing him with a knife. The Carer was shaving the resident who suddenly began to resist intensely and began trying to attack the Carer. The Carer wrote that at this point he deemed it too dangerous to continue the shaving and had to pull back for safety. This Carer is a Polish immigrant and the English language is not his first language. Besides, there is nothing wrong to use the word dangerous to describe a situation you saw first-hand. Had the Carer not recorded the incident, he would be told off. Now he duly recorded the incident, he was also told off. Had the Carer

not attempted to shave the self-neglecting resident, he would also be told off.

3. I walked into a Carer and the nurse in-charge verbally went at each other and I later found out what happened. The Carer made a resident a cup of tea with a plastic cup and the resident spilled some of it on his stomach and a reddish looking discolouration appeared. The nurse became infuriated. The Carer was confronted by the nurse who tried to blame the spill on the fact that a plastic cup instead of ceramic was used to serve the tea as well as the tea temperature not taken prior to serving. The Carer tried to defend herself that the culture of checking tea temperature does not exist and also the plastic cup had a handle and is lighter than ceramic mug so should not be blamed and in trying to get her point across, she asked the nurse why she does not listen. The nurse became furious with the last statement relating to 'listening'. They ended the shift not speaking to each other.

4. A resident who has dementia and could be very anxious and very aggressive or violent lives in our care home. We have tried to manage the risks for such a long while and the only help we got were doctors prescribing calming medication which as I discussed earlier (under stingy Lorazepam), the medication was simply ineffective and the local council completely failed to provide a one-to-one care package for the resident and we were simply told to do half hourly observations to record his whereabout and this particular task was to be done by all Carers who had lots of other tasks to do. One day, we were busy with other tasks and the resident wandered into another resident's bedroom and they had a very bloody fight. All the Carers were told to write a police-like statement stating where they were and what they were doing and basically prove that they were not guilty of failing to stop the violent act. But the local authorities

who did not authorise a one-to-one care package for the resident were not required to also write the same statement. The police interviewed Carers but did not interview the local authority. They didn't interview the doctors who made the calming medication to be attempted only when the resident is obviously and visibly aggressive at which point the resident will likely refuse to take the medication or abuse any Carer who tries to give it to him. The Carers were obviously blamed for the incident. From my perspective and as I have severally highlighted in this memoir, there is that very fast casting of blames on Carers as soon as something goes wrong and it goes up to the point of people considering manslaughter charges against Carers in scenario where a resident choked to death but let's not go that far away from this particular case. The spillage should be blamed on three people.

a. Old age

b. Dementia,

c. Preservation of a resident's independence to drink his tea by himself which has a risk attached.

Do not change the goalpost when something goes wrong like interrogating a Carer why tea temperature was not taken since no one including me even knows if there is a thermometer in the kitchen or where to find it. Besides, who says that serving cold tea to a resident who would rather risk it and have his tea hot as in the concept of mental capacity act is wrong since the resident's care plan did not say serve him cold drinks. The Carer was right and the culture of checking hot food or drinks temperature doesn't exist at that time in that care home and it is not established that the resident's drinks must not be hot for reasons such as regular spilling of drinks.

5. There's a bed-bound resident on two hourly turn/tilt (left, back/bottom and right side) to prevent him from developing

sore bottom on any side due to being on the same side for far too long. The Carers noticed and reported that after each turn/tilt off his bottom, the resident will shuffle himself until he is completely back on his back/bottom against the purpose of the turns/tilt. The management response was to direct the Carers to do the two hourly turns/tilt on a 15 minutes basis with reason being that the first room visit will be for the turn/tilt while the rest of quarter of an hour is to check and tick the box that the resident is actually adhering to.

This made them feel bad because no matter how often the resident is turned, he will always readjust to be on his back/bottom which then translates directly to the Carers turning/tilting him every 15 minutes. The Carers felt they were being blamed and punished for a resident's refusal to adhere to his required/needed treatment which is a prevention treatment in his case and their duty to turn/tilt a man 12 times a 24-hours a day has now become 96 times in every 24 hours and they believe it was because they reported the man's habit of readjusting after each turn since had they not reported the habit, they would not be turning a man 96 times a day. The Carers are unhappy, the resident himself is not happy being disturbed every 15 minutes. Tell me if the Carers will report such habits again if they see it.

Missing items

There is this mysterious way of things going missing in almost all the care homes that I have worked. There are no two ways around it, the culprit is all the people that have been there, and they include Carers, relatives, visitors and other workers at the care home. In the above list of usual suspects, I left out a very serious suspect, residents. Before you attack me for pointing fingers at the residents, read these incidents. I was assisting a male resident to change into pyjamas when searching the pockets to remove paper tissue which ruins clothes in our washing machines, various valuable items fell out. He warned me not to touch them as they were sharp items meant to go in the bins.

Residents should have equal responsibility to build rapport with their Carers. Basic diplomacy, politeness and welcoming body language is a resident's responsibility. I have seen a situation where a resident has been very rude and arrogant towards her Carers when Carers sort of speak to her on strictly official basis and the management attempted to intervene by compelling Carers to go and have a chat with her daily on a more private basis but this intervention was completely futile.

This is the tip of the iceberg and the associated consequences regarding that blame factor where Carers are always at fault taking responsibility for anything and everything. Worst is the feeling of perpetual blame leading to poor learning-from-mistakes, near-miss or mistakes being brushed under the carpet. Recklessly assigning blame or responsibility to Carers means that no one at the top of affairs looked closely at the situation.

The blame factor leads to cover your back syndrome

Things such as the above-mentioned blame factor often lead to Carers preferring to cover their back to solving the problem with a lasting or sustainable solution. It involves stringently avoiding being mentioned in any incident paperwork. It leads to Carers conspiring to brush serious issues under the carpet and deciding to not record incidents as if it never happened. On extreme case, a Carer may witness an incident such as finding a resident on the floor, although it was not his or her fault, that Carer might pretend to not have seen it, walk away and leave the resident on the floor till another Carer sees the resident and then begins the rescue and treatment measures all because if she raised the alarm, she might get interrogated as if she is lying (withholding information) or stressed up or blamed. These are gross misconducts and considerable irresponsibility. The Polish Carer mentioned above, if he were to adopt this system, he would look for any other job that needs doing to do till his shift is over because he knows that trying to shave or wash a self-neglecting resident often leads to an incident report and subsequent interrogation by the local safeguarding team over his English language.

Scapegoating
To protect residents' safety, there must be profound support for Carers working long hours in pressured environments instead of callously scapegoat one Carer who made a mistake and punish the Carer for failures in the system and by so doing discourage Carers from being open to their managers or other safeguarding authorities when reviewing mistakes or shortcomings.

Beg a resident to accept your care service
Residents deserve to receive care services in a dignified manner. Do Carers deserve dignity while giving care?
It is good to adopt a method that works for each resident in order to ensure provision of good quality care service to all residents. Should Carers be expected to lick a resident's ass just because it is a method that works for that resident?
A mentally sound gentleman who had a stroke and his left arm and leg hurt terribly. Carers attend to him, to provide him with personal care in a very careful manner yet, he yells at them and accuses them of torture, and he will be generally rude through his tone and by swearing. They try to explain to him that they weren't the cause of his pain and the fact that he can decline to be turned although consequences may be him developing a bed sore, he agrees to be turned and assisted with personal care but takes it

out on the Carers. In the end, he never appreciates or says thanks. When the Carers go to help him, he thinks they have come to disturb him, then he will appear to think that he is doing them a favour and they should beg him to receive help from them. Some Carers do beg him, plead with him to allow them to provide care. During personal care, he does not help to get turned to his opposite side for his back to be washed or bedsheets removed. When he is asked to put his arm through a clean shirt, he would not even though that he could.

In such a situation or resident, can Carers say, 'do yourself a favour' or 'do me a favour' put this cardigan on because it is a bit cold or have a wash to keep yourself clean? In cases involving residents with reasonable mental capacity, neglects may occur if the resident expects Carers to flatter him/her (especially as if the resident is superior to the Carer) in an obsequious manner, and to support the resident's every opinion and give the resident a lot of attention that is exaggerated and not sincere like fawning over the resident in order to get a positive reaction and for Carers to actually succeed in providing the resident with care. This sort of expectation often causes a fall out between some residents and their Carers and can potentially lead to neglect or residents making false allegations or exaggeration of events especially in situations where it is one resident's words against the resident's Carer's words.

Management's response to allegations
Coroner courts
Let me start this paragraph by quoting a Disneyland Florida advert which says that the 'magic' begins from the moment you tell the kids that they will be going to Disneyland for holiday months before the holiday begins. The psychological torture, on

the other hand, begins the moment you tell Carers that they are being investigated for a resident passing away on their shift.

There are many issues that scare people away from becoming Carers and the possibility of being summoned to coroner court or knowing that deep down you are being listed as suspect manslaughter are major issues. The following event occurred, and I am not narrating it to discourage investigation into unexpected deaths. I am rather of the opinion that such must not be reckless, and care must be taken to not make such inquiry or investigation seem like a hanging noose on the neck of Carers for months in each event of unexpected death. It must be quick and any Carer who has absolutely nothing to do with it should be completely removed from it. Carers want to do their job, go home, rest and have their peace of mind remaining undisturbed. News I heard that my colleagues have a coroner court to attend with regards to the death of one of the residents caused each one of us to reconsider the job (working in care). My colleagues started a night shift at 8pm, did the first round of checks after their handover around 8:30 pm. They began the next round of checks at 10pm and found a lady had passed away on getting to her room before 11pm. Before you read any further, do understand that Carers are not doctors & to detect the internal state of someone's body during such hourly or bi-hourly room checks to know whether a resident is in critical condition or to differentiate between hearing a snoring or breathing that may sound congested, like a rattle or gurgle which possibly indicates that someone may be dying will obviously remain a challenge to Carers. Now, the GP refused to sign the death certificate because she was not seen by her own GP in preceding 2 weeks before her death so her death was classed as suspicious despite her long list of medical conditions which include stroke, being fed through her stomach with a tube, etc. All the Carers on the shift were phoned and informed that they will be attending a coroner court. They were also informed that failure to attend may warrant an arrest. This coroner court and issues will be concluded in the next six months so Carers who are a layman in terms of law and so forth will have to spend the next six months worrying. Even though it was not their responsibility to arrange a GP visit, the death of the resident has put them under investigation, and they will be interviewed or interrogated. This phone call to inform them upset the Carers. They go through all these for minimum wage (living wage). Who else would like to do the job? Looking after vulnerable people presents a considerable amount of risk of mistakes happening. One mistake or one error of judgement could land a Carer in jail on a manslaughter charge. Working in a warehouse or food manufacturing or supermarket will get one the same living wage but with zero chance of worrying over anything like manslaughter charges or such.

Carers are not paid well enough to absorb reckless 'manslaughter' charges, sort of risk or rope being hanging on their neck or be attached to the job role. Carers are mostly below college education. Most of them are equally not educated enough on how to protect themselves in certain intricate situations and defend themselves legally and they are not paid enough to keep a permanent 'conciliar' (legal advisor) as you'd expect someone who is in a seriously risky business would have.

Suspended pending investigation

To avoid inevitable neglect that results from Carers' fear of 'suspension-pending-investigation' outcome, management and relatives must begin a proactive reassurance of all care staff to not be afraid of providing personal care to such residents who resort to allegations and threats of false allegations. Let the Carers know this. Formally reassure all staff. Remember suspension pending investigation outcome is on its own punishment for doing no wrong and a good care team is all out for one of their team members and one for all, punishment for one who has done no wrong is punishment for all and neglect of such resident who make false alarm due to fear of victimisation is inevitably guaranteed.

According to the Guardian 1st December 2017, "Hundreds of mourners have lined the streets of a tiny Welsh town for the funeral of the former Welsh Labour minister Carl Sargeant, who was eulogised as "kindness in a big bundle". The 49-year-old was found having taken his own life at his home on 7 November, four days after being sacked from his role as cabinet secretary for communities and children amid allegations of harassment"

Allegations are very powerful and powerful enough to cause an individual to take or consider taking their own life. But one thing that is more powerful than allegations is False allegations. Even if made by a mentally challenged individual, it is still more powerful than ordinary allegations. Most residents hate to live in care homes. The idea scares most of them. They want their children to take them home. And if they are tricked into staying in a care home on respite with the intention of making it permanent, some residents attempt most dubious means to achieve one particular objective which is to go home and not live in a care home. One of such dubious means is to exaggerate incidents, make allegations and exhibit serious inappropriate behaviours. Relatives are vulnerable because they trust their elderly relative very well and therefore easily convinced that whatever they hear is the absolute truth. Just bear the above in mind while dealing with any incidents, allegations, and serious inappropriate behaviours. If the suspension is inevitable then adequate reassurance must be put in place to at least reduce the psychological burden that the staff involved may experience during the investigation period which should be made haste. Managers, on the other hand, must start to validate all allegations before the suspension of suspects pending a full investigation.

Allegations are an as powerful predicament as imaginable and till today, the biggest killer of compassionate care. Let us look at an allegation of a paedophile that was made against Sir Cliff Richard. In August 2014, police raided his home following the allegations which were that he had abused boys between 1958 and 1983 but at the end of the investigation, he was never charged. Still, Cliff Richard doubts he will ever recover from the abuse allegations.

According to him during an interview with ITV on 18th July 2018, years after he was exonerated,
"Sir Cliff on the impact of the case has had on him
Referring to the past three years as "turmoil" he said the allegations made against him had had a significant impact on him and his behaviour.
He said: "I'm sure I'll recover [from this]. There are aspects in my life that I recognise now. For instance, at Wimbledon there is a tunnel between Centre Court and Court One, I used to use it regularly to see the matches I was interested in on Court One. And it went right past the ball boys' dressing room. I will not go there now.
"I won't go anywhere near children...even when I'm having photographs taken, I try not to make contact. It has taken something away from me."
When this sort of thing happens in care towards a Carer, the relationship will be finished, rebuilding such relationships will not start from ground zero, it will rather start from ground minus one hundred. A Carer may dread walking past a corridor due to allegations.

Allegations (pointing fingers)

A resident who has dementia was looking for his eyeglasses as he sat down with his visiting relatives in the lounge. The relatives reported to the day's senior who herself asked all day Carers on shift and was told that the resident who was earlier in the morning, washed and dressed by night Carers didn't come out of his bedroom to the lounge/dining room wearing the glasses earlier in the morning of that day. Later, when the night team arrived for another night shift, the senior interrupted the night team's handover to ask the night Carer about the glasses and she responded that the resident had it on when he came out. Later, as I was cleaning the lounge chairs, I found the missing glasses in between chair's arm and chair's cushion where the resident sat. The Carer involved became tearful and I realised she was hurt badly when I told her where I found the glasses. She then told me that when she opened the door to let the relatives out when they were leaving, one of them said to her exactly what the senior said that the night Carers didn't put on his glasses earlier in the day. She was very upset because she was blamed for the glasses missing. She felt betrayed in some way and felt like she was called a liar as everyone alleged that she lost the glasses in another way. Allegations are far too powerful than people imagine and what is worse is false allegations. I was attending to a resident who is renowned for reporting his Carers to the management on a regular basis. He was happy with me and we were having a lovely conversation in a very happy mood. Suddenly, he asked me for my name. I felt a shock and I asked why he wanted to know my name and in a fake smile I tried to laugh it off that he knows my name already and challenged him to remember. I did not feel like telling him my name is the fact. I was afraid of doing so because he was renowned for trying to put Carers into unnecessary trouble. At the end I told him I am his Carer. My reason for including this is to show how Carers do certain things like distancing themselves from residents out of fear.

Residents, Carers and management should never overreact by making false or wrong allegations. Allegations are very serious matters even in the outside world. For instance, in June 2019, former Celebrity Big Brother contestant Roxanne Pallett was told she was "more hated than a murderer" after falsely accusing her fellow housemate, Ryan Thomas of physically assaulting her during the live show which was viewed live by millions of people. The public condemnation was overwhelming. Media watchdog OFCOM received 11,215 complaints over the episode and she later issued an apology and said she had "overreacted".

Most false allegations may be over-reaction but then once the falsehood has gathered momentum, it will be very difficult to not hurt or upset someone or a group of people.

If any Carer or resident and/or the management have made this 'over-reaction' mistake, the quicker an apology is issued, the better and smoother the healing process. Refusing to apologise due to big ego or arrogance will be like fanning the flame.

Male Carers 'out of bounds'

Male Carers are very good Carers. They are patient, caring and have as much right to work in the care industry as nurses and doctors and females. If you are uncomfortable with a male Carer, then indicate at the admission stage the same time when you disclose your preferences and allergy. I must suggest that the management and relatives do ask this particular question to all residents at assessment and have their preference respected because some residents have voiced their preference in most ridiculous ways by making false allegations against male Carers and in some cases, the male Carer accused was not even on the shift. There was a lady on the other hand who was alright with female Carers or male Carers assisting her with personal care. One night, she insisted that she must have only male Carers. All female Carers agreed with her request and their point was since some female residents were granted their preference to receive personal care from only a female Carer, this lady's preference should be allowed. The male Carers disagreed, their point was that they were not "gigolo" and queried why she would smile at them or wink her eye at them male Carers and now her preference must be disallowed and if she was not going to allow a female Carer assist her with personal care, she will not be assisted by either of them ever again. A serious dilemma arose. This dilemma.

The stereotypes and challenges that men face are not to be ignored. The fact is that the industry needs more human resources; hence, not in a position to pick and choose a gender. It is wrong to say no more male doctors required and equally wrong to abuse male Carers for their gender. I was once told by an angry female resident, "no one will ever have you help; you should not be working here, you are useless". She angrily said all that to me because I told her that other female Carers were busy and since she will not let me (a male Carer) assist her, she needs to wait a little longer for my female colleagues. She got angry and said those words because she believed that my being on the shift somehow delayed her receiving care from a female Carer since the other female Carer on shift were busy assisting someone else and she only prefers female Carers and the management won't because of me or her increasing the number of staff. There were 2 female Carers and one male Carer (me) on that night shift.

On another night, a female resident hesitantly agreed to allow a male Carer to assist with her washing after an experienced female Carer had spoken to her, perhaps persuaded or encouraged the resident to. The funny, rather serious thing was that the female Carer after speaking to the resident went to the male Carer and advised him to 'be cordial and diplomatic and most importantly to be careful and avoid lingering while cleaning the resident' s private area. This is the most upsetting and equally stupid thing I ever have heard. If there is a high risk of the resident making allegations of such serious nature as saying that the male Carer lingered while cleaning her, then why put the Carer in such a position in the first place?

Lack of common sense is like an affliction rooting up to the marrow of the industry. Another good example is this rule or stipulation which prevents two male Carers from assisting a resident (who requires a couple of Carers) with personal care because they are two males but not because the resident has made prior 'out of bound male Carers' demand. Besides, a male Carer working with a female Carer is totally acceptable to assist female residents. But consider that one male Carer can assist any female resident who has not made prior 'out of bound male Carers' demand but two male Carers cannot. Could it not be classified as another issue of sexism since two female Carers are totally acceptable to assist a male resident who has not made prior 'out of bound female Carers' demand. Where exactly is the sense?

A male Carer in the female-dominated team is the odd one who sometimes must put up with the perception as being expendable. In some manoeuvre situations where risk of back injury is likely, he will be expected to be strong and on his own, lift heavy residents or wash residents who have been assessed to require two staff for such manoeuvre due to the risk or be told by other female things like, 'I can even do him/her by myself'. If the cartons of deliveries arrive, he will be the first person to be assigned the duty of carrying the boxes to the storage room or he will be the first person to be blamed should the boxes be left at the entrance for long. The ladies will sometimes make him the subject of their discussion more of gossip in a very disrespectful manner and if he walks into the discussion, the rest of the team goes mum. If the manager thinks that the shift is overstaffed and wants one Carer to go to the sister-care home who may be running short staffed, the male Carer is twice as likely to be asked to go.

Most violent residents will be allocated to the male Carer to stay with on a one-to-one basis until the resident calms down probably because of the assumption that male Carer can better withstand verbal or physical abuse. If very obese residents need to go to the hospital, a male Carer is first to be asked to go with the resident because it is assumed, he is better at pushing a wheelchair. A bed needs moving from one room to another, he will be asked. The care industry really needs to change this mindset and attitude towards male Carers or else there will be fewer of them joining in.

Bruises on residents

The most prevalent source of bruises on residents' bodies is the residents own fingernails and toenails. Residents use their toenail to scratch their other leg or foot or/and using their fingernails to scratch their bodies. Residents scratch due to itchy feeling.

It is very unfortunate that such a stereotype or prejudice exists such that whenever a bruise is found on a resident, the first assumption would be that Carers did it. The assumption that Carers did it by being too rough or less careful. Although in some cases, this stereotype is correct just like a dead clock being correct twice each day. It is also necessary to keep in mind that residents do regularly ask Carers to scratch their bodies for them. A gentleman requested that I 'scratch his back' and I responded that, I am so sorry sir, but I cannot do that for you. I can assist you to have a shower or apply ointment to your skin, but I will not scratch your back or any other part of your body. If I do that and bruise your body in the process, I would be done for it. The gentleman got angry with me and asked me to fetch someone else who would scratch for him.

Elbow/arm bruises may be caused by squeezing tight clothes especially shirts on residents
The major cause of wrist bruises is bad handling of residents especially residents who have Deprivation of liberty safeguards (DOLS) in place for being resistive but the next major cause is metallic wrist watches and bangles.
Pant line and groin marks/bruises
Pants for residents should be able to hold the pad in place firmly but should not make a round red-grip-mark on both laps or groin and/or on the resident's hip/belt area. The reinforced elasticated edges of pants and socks too make it tight enough to cause bruises or red marks so I suggest that just as I said earlier regarding socks, three thin cuts be made on the elasticated edges to weaken the grip on laps and hip.
Flannels cause bruises. There are different qualities of flannel range and you can bet care homes purchase the cheapest of all which is the lowest quality. After a long time of use, its fluffy soft bits wear out and it becomes frictional especially with hard water. It is advisable that Carers wash residents with soaked wet wipes instead of wet flannels unless the flannel is a soft gentle one.

Double-padding
'Double-padding' is simply a practice of putting two sanitary pads on the resident at the same time and is a form of abuse.
Let us look at this text message,

"Hi please be aware that the wrap around pads are only for JH, WK and AL. And the pull ups are only for JB and VK. Please do not use these pads for any other residents as this is why we keep running out. Thanks"

A case of a male resident with about 7inches sized penis who was issued with an 'always ultra' (5 inches wide by 10 inches long) size pad. staff must take what they consider to be the appropriate pad from another resident to give to this man. In other words, Carers improvise when they do not get what they need. To understand it, you must separate 'need' from 'want' and it is not what they want, rather, it is what they really need. Take, for instance, Carers use quilt/duvet cover in place of bedsheets when the care home has a very low or zero number of washed/dried bedsheets. Carers also put fitted bed sheets on air mattresses against best practice advice when they have little or no non-fitted bed sheets. No one notices or cares because doing either of the above is not classed as abuse. Also, no one notices when they wear double gloves due to being given poor quality vinyl gloves that rip in the middle of personal care. Neither of these was classed as abuse. The only reason anyone noticed that Carers are 'taking' other residents' pads to give on another resident was because they were running out faster than they were supposed to.

The wrap around pads are considered by Carers to be the best quality. Unfortunately, this quality pad is not for everyone.

The following text messages came from just one care home in a space of five months:

"Hi please be aware that the wrap around pads are only for JH, WK and AL. And the pull ups are only for JB and VK. Please do not use these pads for any other residents as this is why we keep running out. Laura.

Thanks"

"Hi all the pull up pads are only to be used for JB and VK. The wrap around pads are only to be used for WK, AL and JH. Do not use these pads for any other residents. Thanks"

"Please note RC and JH are the only residents that use the wrap around pads. Thanks"

"All staff must not be using wrap around pads except for J and R pls Thanks"

These messages indicate that the motive for using the high-quality wrap around pad on a resident who it was not meant for was not deemed a serious issue or an abuse. However, the same motive applies to double padding.

Another good scenario to describe double padding for your understanding is your vehicle which requires a tube and a tyre but due to inadequate funds, you gave your mechanic one tube and another tube to reserve for you while not providing your mechanic with a tyre which is needed. Your mechanic installs one tube but realises that the vehicle cannot even run on one tube without outer tyre so decides to add the reserve tube that you provided to improvise and get you from point A to B. Residents need the pad to prevent them getting soaked in a pool of their own urine and affecting their dignity. The best practice is to believe Carers when they report that a resident is losing his or her continence and believe Carers if they report that the wrong incontinence pad has been provided since it does too little or nothing to help with a resident's heavy flow or that the little pad you provided is not a good fit for the resident, therefore, it is ineffective. Assess residents who Carers report has appeared to lose their continent. The pad is given to them at bedtime and to be checked at pre-set intervals and if wet, then changed. The interval may be 2 hourly checks or 4 hourlies in some care homes. The pad is supposed to stop the urine spreading to soak the resident's body and pyjamas or nightdress or day clothes and hold the urine till the next check is done and the pad is changed and a fresh pad put in place. Due to underfunding of the industry, the NHS puts residents on waiting list, sometimes the incontinent team do not believe Carers who report that a resident is incontinent and many months later when the pads finally arrive, the wrong pad is sent to the resident, you realise that the resident still gets soaking wet up to the bedsheet and night dresses every time that he/she becomes incontinent in between the stipulated 2 hourly checks to the point that the bed sheets and duvets would need to be changed and sometimes up to thrice in a night. This is a fact. Carers who put double pads mostly do it to prevent and protect that sort of soaking. The ideal thing is to contact the NHS for a reassessment of incontinence but this often fact fully results in months of waiting as well as them requesting for the wet pads to be kept and stored for them because they assume the Carers are lying. This is still part of providing Carers with their necessary supplies. I once saw a 'digni-TEA' party poster next to a resident's bedroom whom I had assisted up and had been reporting to the seniors that he needs a proper pad as the tiny sized pad given to him is unable to serve the purpose. What dignity do we celebrate when residents are bedwetting daily?

Double padding residents is a serious abuse and should result in dismissal but a different approach should be adopted to stop it such as looking into whether the resident needs a much bigger absorbing pad or checking if the resident gets soaked from one check to the next check during the night. The fact that there is a difference between pads designated for the daytime and pads designated for the night-time is a clear indication of the variety of expectations and situations with time. The large absorbing green pads are provided for night-time because the alternative purple or grey pads are deemed inadequate or ineffective to serve the resident at night. This assessment may sound basic, but it is very critical. When the management provides an inadequate or ineffective pad to a resident, the outcome is usually "double padding" unless a very exceptionally strict Carer is around to stop his or her colleagues from doing so. This is prevalent in badly run care homes.

Abuse is abuse, Rape is rape
If a resident with dementia grabs a Carer by his or her genitals, the psychological impact is no different if the same act was done by an individual without dementia outside a care home. On the other hand, if a mentally sound individual sexually assaults a Carer outside a care home, the psychological impact is no different if the same act was done by an individual with mental health issues within a care home. It should be treated as such. An adequate disclosure must be made by relatives, the resident's previous care homes and other institutions who have in their possession any sexually inappropriate behaviour record of any resident to the new care home that is admitting that resident during the admission stage and Carers must be protected from abuse of all forms.

As part of the resident's admission orientation I suggested, it will be good to explain to residents about how serious Sexual abuse or harassment is taken, what constitute Sexual harassment and how to not get into trouble.

Let me share one instance out of many, a male resident who has a condom catheter which 'comes off' on its own thrice in an hour. The first time, a male Carer (me) went and simply fixed a fresh condom catheter for him and while leaving his room, the resident asked after a female Carer and sent his regards. The second time the female Carer fixed it for him. The third time I went again and as I walked in, he wasn't very happy that I came so he asked if I could send the female Carer instead, I declined and informed him that he risk running out before he received his next monthly supply of condom catheter and he denied any knowledge of reasons behind it regularly 'coming off'. I suspect that he kept taking it out hoping that the female Carer will come back, hold his sex organ to re-affix a fresh condom catheter. Isn't this a clear instant of Sexual Harassment at work?

Abuse of Carers
Is it or should it be the Carers responsibility to receive degrading gestures and any form of abuse from a resident without mental capacity or/and from a resident with full mental capacity even if there is a good chance of successfully completing the objectives of meeting the resident's care needs by allowing such gestures? Do the following United Nations' fundamental human rights which guarantees everyone rights exclude Carers?

"Article 1.
All human beings are born free and equal in dignity and rights. They are endowed with reason and conscience and should act towards one another in a spirit of brotherhood.

Article 5.
No one shall be subjected to torture or to cruel, inhuman or degrading treatment or punishment"

As clear as it is, Lord Janner was alleged to have abused vulnerable children but unfit to plead or stand trial due to his mental health state. Most elderly people are suffering from dementia or have other medical conditions which would make them unable to plead. This does not mean if a male resident with dementia grabs his Carer at her bottom or genital such Carer would not feel the same psychological burden felt by rape victims. This is an everyday issue in many care homes today. The big problem is that when a man suffering from dementia exhibits this behaviour, most female Carers are scared of coming forward to report it and in some instances where the man involved moves to another care home, his relatives often withhold to mention and warn the new care home to put adequate measures in place to protect the staff.

A situation fast developing is one which Carers who are sexually assaulted or who witnessed a resident get sexually assaulted do not come forward and the reason is not because of shame feeling but because they have been subconsciously embedded with the idea that nothing can be done or will be done about it and/or the attacker is suffering dementia therefore lacking premeditated motive so it should be classed as collateral damage. Unfortunately, this goes on and on until a pure clear rape incident takes place and then the management is forced to take extreme action.

Response to attack of care staff

On 20th March 2019, the BBC reported that Southampton General Hospital Accident and Emergency department Security staff at Southampton General Hospital's A&E department's Security staff voted for a series of strikes over lack of protective equipment and inadequate payments for staff injured at work.

They said that they were being attacked on members of the public, either under the influ drugs or with mental health problems.

They are asking for personal protection gear suc and safety restraints, six months' full pay followed t half-pay for all sickness absences as well as investigations" into any attacks. Now think of it this w. hospitals have security to protect them, but care homes do n Any such attacks by members of the public, either under the influence of drink or drugs, or residents with mental health problems may successfully land on the Carers who are not protected. Whatever is granted to the Hospital Security staff should be made law and granted to Carers also. Carers in care homes are too neglected to speak out and yet they undergo exact same abuse.

NHS Care homes care plan data sharing

ABC notes could be symptoms of a medical condition so should be reported to be on NHS database

All daily notes, assessments, and recordings including ABC of serious cases should be kept in the NHS database for Long-term availability and use. Care home policies of holding on to such folders and destroying them after 3 years {sometimes less} puts Carers at risk when such individuals are transferred from their care home to another and certain pieces of information are not passed on and that individual's assessment becomes inaccurate leading to risk of abuse of either Carers or the individual.

Should Care Homes Have CCTV

Installation of CCTV cameras in care homes should be encouraged by all. Abuse in care homes is two-way traffic. In one way, Carers are often the victim of abuse perpetrated by 's visitors, management and residents themselves while ~~~~ other way, residents are the victims of abuse perpetrated ~~~~ esident's visitors, management, fellow residents and Carers. ~~~~ e only issue Carers have is that the cameras are fixed to capture ONLY abuses toward the elderly residents, aimed at catching Carers in the act and aimed at preventing the abuse of all elderly residents who live in the care home but will not be aimed at capturing verbal, sexual, physical, psychological and emotional abuse of Carers by the elderly residents (most of whom will be deemed unable to enter any plea in court just like Lord Jenner), relatives of elderly residents and the care home management who will not abide by the best practice of Human resource management. Cameras in care homes will in my personal prediction capture the abuses against Carers as listed above in over 90% of the time but the police and management and society at large would deem such abuses as collateral damage and expect the Carers to bear the burden and carry on as if it didn't happen but then the consequences of bearing such burden will result in abused Carers deliberately or not deliberately neglecting a resident or other form of abuse toward a resident by a Carer (who snapped) in 10% of the time and then it will be reported all over the news media that a Carer was caught in the act. The only time the public realised that installing cameras in all classrooms would capture lots of images of students abusing teachers and little images of teachers abusing students were after teachers were stabbed by their students and one of the teachers died of the stab wound.

The people who will suffer most if cameras are installed together with compulsory compensation for any abused Carer are the insurance companies because for example; any Carer groped by a resident who is too old or medically unfit to enter a plea in court can have the camera evidence and claim compensation for the abuse suffered which will be payable within coverage of the care home's public liability insurance policy. The camera will lay bare the abuses that Carers suffer. It will show how tiny the elevator really is for a pregnant Carer and a resident in a wheelchair to fit into. The level of claim will be so high that they will be forced to remove the cameras and the debate over why should cameras be installed will shift toward why should a Carer's fundamental human rights to live including the right to work in the care industry free of any form of abuse be ignored. Installing cameras will show us that, the public liability insurance has not been covering the Carers until cameras are installed. The premium will skyrocket to astonishing new rates and this new bill will be collected by care homes and subsequently added to the amount being charged to residents and local authorities and this will lead to further debate on either local authorities lift any lid on highest amount payable per resident or care homes will choose to shut down their businesses.

Cameras will lay bare all that is written in this memoir.

With the insurance premium rising up with the continued exposure of the abuse of Carers and subsequent compensation claims, care homes will be cherry picking which resident they admit and any resident with a record of abuse toward his or her Carers will not be easily accepted.

On 8th February 2017, ITV reported, 'Teachers using body-cameras in a trial to combat unruly pupils'. Teachers who are beginning to wear a body camera to deter pupils from behaving badly and to record exact behaviour. Police wear cameras too one of their reasons is to protect both policemen and the public. NHS staff wear a body camera and that is not new. The only other group who have not tried body cameras are the Carers. If you suspect foul play, install a camera. The camera is welcomed since it is unbiased. You must be ready to welcome whatever feedback camera brings which may not be what you are expecting to see. Personally, from experience, residents abuse Carers on a larger scale than Carers abuse residents. The only difference is it is institutionalised that abuse of Carers is seen as normal and acceptable because elderly people are deemed as vulnerable adults and above the law in most cases.

Response to bad behaviours

The only existing thing that Carers are expected to do when a resident behaviour is simply unacceptable is to document it. This simply did not address the issue of what to do or how to react at that point in time. Carers are human beings who have feelings. This poor clarity leads to Carers reacting differently sometimes right and sometimes wrong. Here are a few moments that I noted when they happened. I do not know if I am right or wrong. You judge.

Forced Interaction is not the key

"stop watching TV, interact with the residents". In some Care homes when Carers' relationship breakdown, their interaction with the residents suffers as well. But the management often fail to investigate the reasons behind this and would attempt to force interactions without resolving whatever had broken it in the first place.

I have worked on a day shift where the manager switches the TV off and asks the Carers to interact with the residents. Even if there is not any breakdown of relationship, Carers need conversation triggers, something to discuss over and about. A good TV programme can help if it is interesting enough. But then forcing interactions is an authoritarian style and is not the right approach. Promoting a happier environment will achieve that. Trying to find out why Carers interact and why sometimes they do not interact much with residents should have been the first thing to observe.

Manners costs nothing

I pushed the hot drinks trolley into the lounge to serve residents starting from the entrance end and in turn by turn basis. There is this very impatient resident who as soon as she sees the trolley, she wants to be served first so she starts shouting at me for tea and then gets louder and louder. I usually feel bad about her behaviour mainly because she has full capacity and knows exactly what she is doing. I reacted to it by continuing to serve on turn by turn basis and making sure she served last by skipping her when I got to her turn. Then I brought the next round of drinks later in the shift about a couple of hours later and she was so quiet and composed so I served her first and she smiled. The idea of playing into bad behaviour is wrong in my very own opinion.

Refusing to be branded 'tea man' right or wrong?

I am usually the most likely Carer to make residents drink when I am on shift. But this provokes an unfortunate reaction from some residents without sound manners. For instance, when one resident sees me, whether busy or not, she remembers one thing, 'tea' and she will shout at me to make her a cup of tea. This went on to an extent that she was having a chat with another Carer but the moment she saw me walking through the door she shouted at me, can I have a cup of tea and then turned to a resident next to her and told her that I am the tea man. This behaviour on the contrary did not make me want to make her a cuppa at that moment.   I   did   not   like   that.
I arrived at work and went to say hello to residents in the lounge. Each resident acknowledged and asked how I was. One other resident could not stop shouting at me, 'my Horlicks' over and

over again so I went closer to her ears and whispered, 'when a Carer arrives and comes to you and greets you, you ask how they are rather than be shouting for Horlicks over and over' and she said, 'oh I'm sorry'.

Warning a resident to stop swearing at you or not receive your assistance, right or wrong?

I was assisting a resident to use her Commode and she kept swearing and saying things like, 'what a bloody game this is' and I said to her politely, if you swear one more time I will suspend assisting you any further and get out of your room. I am not swearing, am I? if I am not swearing while I am here in your room then you must not be swearing while I am here helping you. A resident pressed the call bell for assistance, and I responded, as I knocked on the door and walked in, we made eye contact and I greeted her. She totally looked away in a body language that simply said that she was not pleased to see me and totally ignored me. Then I said well if you don't want to be assisted by me, then I will go and you can press the bell again to have someone else, but I will record and report your behaviour, she then spoke to me about what she wanted which she said she would rather have someone else due to me being male Carer.

Attention seeking

Attention seeking is a very serious problem which Carers face. It occurs in various ways, most of which are challenging behaviours such as a resident constantly shouting. In this care home, a resident is fond of a Carer. Once she notices that the Carer has started her shift, give it a few minutes and she will start shouting for that particular Carer to attend to her and soon after that she will start shouting again that This behaviour begins about a quarter past eight in the night and perfectly correlates with the night shift Carer's prompt eight start of shift and the resident usually has a nose bleed as soon as she begins shouting the Carer's name. At the beginning, we did not know what was going on, so we very much played into it. The resident had a clip to hold her nose by firmly pinching the soft part of her nose and it effectively stopped the bleeding, but she kept removing the clip before the bleeding stopped. In order to prevent her from prematurely removing the clip, we asked the Carer she was fond of to sit down with her in her room but as soon as the Carer goes, the bleeding restarts. The Carer ended up staying with her on one to one basis most of the night. On another night, when the bleeding had gone on for an uncomfortable long, we had to inform her that we were calling ambulance service and it was very necessary that she got ready to go to the hospital with them if they didn't stop the bleeding or needed to check the cause. She clearly told us that she does not want to go to the hospital. The bleeding which had gone unstoppable on and off for a few hours suddenly stopped completely. We were happy but when this same story began to happen over and over in the exact same order and in a timely manner, a pattern was well noted. We noticed a pattern developing after too many coincidences which were recorded. We also noted that telling her that she risked going to the hospital stops the nosebleed quicker than sending her the Carer whose name she was shouting nonstop before and during every nosebleed episode.

Call bell monitoring for checking misuse

Take, for instance, abuse of antibiotics guarantees that taking antibiotics will no longer guarantee anyone a complete recovery from bacterial infection. Abuse of call bell on the other hand by one resident leads to a delayed response to other residents with genuine needs and neglect of other residents who do not or cannot use the call bell.

The best way to describe call bell misuse, on the other hand, is a situation where my resident was being assisted with personal care in his bed by two Carers, he saw the call bell system and reached to it and pressed it. This particular resident is renowned for misusing the call bell by everyone including seniors but no report has been filed and no action has been taken but when Carers asked him why he pressed the call bell since we were already with him providing care to him, he simply said he didn't know. So, it appears that the call bell system can indeed be misused. Similarly, a situation arose where my resident has risk of falls while in his bedroom so a floor sensor mat was installed on the floor next to his bed so that a Carer will dash to his room each time to stop him falling but then there were many times when he did not want to stand up and didn't want to lay down, instead he just wanted to sit up with his foot on the sensor floor mat for a while. This makes the mat continue to trigger over and over which makes the Carers dash to his room over and over which then stresses up the Carers. These issues exist in all care homes and even paramedics have similar issues too.

Now, let us review this text message,

"Morning all, polite request to pls ensure we support one another at night. We're one home let's work together. Also, call bells/mats are never to be unplugged. If someone is getting up a lot etc then pls document it or ABC it as currently the concerns raised are not reflected in charts. Thanks for your support

Thanks"

This message did say document the situation but it did not say what to do at that particular time when the problem was ongoing and how to respond to the problem rather than unplugging/disabling that individual's call bell or sensor mat. Also, the text didn't advise what to do in terms of staffing level since a member of staff has to be assigned or dedicated to answering the call bells or sensor floor mat calls of one particular resident over and over in complete detriment of other residents. The text did not say how soon the documents (if documented) will be reviewed and relevant action taken in line with the increased need or increased attention seeking.

To check abuse or misuse of the call bell system and ensure fairness in terms of providing rational and adequate attention to all the residents rather than the ones who regularly and perpetually sought Carers' attention at the detriment of the ones that did not or could not. This is the most sensitive issue to write about because there is a considerable thin line between ignoring someone who very often cries wolf and justifying your reasons for not taking the blame and responsibility should the same person get eaten by a real wolf at some point in the future. Regularly pressing the call bell which makes Carers run and if done for no good reason causes a lot of hurt and damages genuine compassionate care. It is a pointless warning that regularly crying wolf when there was not any wolf is dangerous; hence, something must be done. I worked at this care home that provided call bell forms for monitoring purposes. Before I begin, let first clarify that there are numerous ways for Carers to remotely get a hint of where they are needed to be or who they need to attend to such includes the wall call bell, floor sensors, pendant call bells, movement sensors etc but the most abused of all these is the call bells. A resident pressing the call bell for a Carer to come and assist that resident to do a task that the resident can very easily do by herself. A gentleman complained about his neighbour receiving Carers' attention every time and he saw the Carers walk past his bedroom and he said it because he rarely pressed the call bell, unlike his neighbour who pressed it all the time. Another true story was a gentleman who was bed bound keeps his call bell trigger under his body and it goes off each time he turns on the bed. A Carer would respond whenever it goes off ringing and the gentleman will not know what he wanted and claimed he did not call. After some calls, one of the Carers told the gentleman in a firm voice to buzz only when he needs assistance. Another Carer overheard this and reported it to the manager who furiously questioned the Carer for daring to tell residents when to and when not to press the call bell. Now you can see that the issue relating to call bell misuse has caused a problem between two Carer's relationships with each other. You cannot expect those two Carers to work together and make good teammates for the rest of that shift or day, would you? Later, after a few more calls from the gentleman, Carers went to change his pad and then discovered why the call was going off nonstop, the resident was laying down on the call bell switch. There should be a way of identifying abuse of the call bell system and preventing it. I would limit my suggestion to the fact that this prevention of abuse certainly begins with identifying residents who have been reported by different Carers for pressing the call bell unnecessarily and strictly recording whatever the reasons and whenever that resident presses the call bell, analysing the records of that residents calls as recorded by responding Carer and discussing with the resident's relative to proffer a solution, one that will also provide a safeguard for the residents while at the same time preventing abuse of the call bell system and other unfairness that goes with it. Managers should understand that it is critically important to clearly explain to Carers how to react to these problems before the situation arises because not knowing what to do or expecting the Carers to absorb the stress that comes from the call bell abuse or misuse hasn't worked. A half an hour observations schedule for some residents could be an alternative in some cases if the call bell is being regularly misused. Other

Call bell Palaver
It is a very bad thing for any resident to dread using the call bell. It is, in fact, a serious abuse for any Carer to tell a resident that they are pressing the call bell too much or tell the resident not to press the call bell at all. Having highlighted that, there is a need to look into situations where Carers get frustrated because a resident is misusing the call bell which results in shifting Carers attention from other residents in the care home and giving it to the one pressing the call bell regularly.

Lack of fair-use-of-call bell policy is discriminatory to residents who cannot or would not use the call bell
Biggest residents' competition in a care home is to attract the attention of the Carers. Unfortunately, the staffing levels of care homes reflect the profitability mindset of the investors thereby requiring Carers to divide their attention among all the residents making 'attention' a limited rationed service. The problem emerges when some residents are not satisfied with their allotted fair share of the attention that the Carers could possibly give in order to be fair to other residents. Some residents have call bells and are able to use it to call for the attention of Carers and Carers must respond to see what help the resident needs. Some other residents do not have the capacity to use the call bell, so they do not have any means or capacity to request Carers attention for their own needs. The use of 'targets' by management to monitor average response time to call bells by Carers does indirectly give priority for more attention, checks and care to be provided to residents who can press the call bell against those who cannot.

In various instances, Carers in the middle of personal care have to pause to run and respond to the call bell of another resident who has only just been assisted with care by them and sometimes more frustratingly this same resident would seek their attention over and over again whilst they are in the process of helping other residents. This unfair disadvantage is heightened when there is no mechanism in place to curb or monitor very clear abuse of the call bell system whether knowingly or unknowingly, whether purposely or not by residents who can press the call bell. The sensitivity surrounding the call bell means that Carers dare not complain or speak out against a call-bell misuse for fear of being deemed 'abusive toward residents' and this is as a matter of fact the prevalent ideal and the result of not having a right path to address call bell misuse often leads to Carers lashing out at a resident they deem to have been abusing the call bell or disconnect the call bell for a while either of which remains acts which will then be classed as abuse. Carers dare not say to a resident not to use the call bell at such critical/busy times and they dare not disconnect the call bell either these two actions warrant immediate sack as a disciplinary action.

Newton's law
Every action, there is an equal and opposite reaction
In quoting this law of physics, critics would jump straight into conclusions that I am insinuating that a deliberate tit-for-tat or eye for an eye would occur whenever a Carer gets abused or maltreated either by residents, relatives or management. Of course not! The reaction differs significantly, not completely or in exact form or shape. This law applies to humanity and our behaviour towards one another. No Carer or any health care worker or professional will ever tell you this or agree to its reality or existence since doing so may suggest to people that the person

may retaliate should a vulnerable service user abuse him or her. A Carer or a mother who has been abused (a Carer who just been slapped or spat in the face) by her resident or child would react naturally but in different ways to the abuse received. If you beat a child, the child may react by crying. On the other hand, if a resident in a grumpy way requests for assistance, it often leads to service without any smile and on a more serious instance, it may lead to the ruining of the Carer's day or mood and being in a bad mood may lead to working in a non-compassionate manner or providing service without a smile throughout the Carer's shift on that particular day or night and beyond it can affect the relationship between the Carer and the grumpy residents. Although this may not be considered as abuse at a safe level anything less than compassionate care is unacceptable and on advanced levels, a bad mood can actually lead to preventable accidents or even an abuse taking place most prevalent being verbal abuse like swearing in a murmuring tone. Similarly, a resident abusing the call bell system could lead to the Carers naturally feeling reluctant to respond in line with the 'crying of wolf' parable.

This memoir is not condoning the abuse of residents or defending any Carer who is or has abused a resident. Contrary to that, this memoir attempts to identify various mostly undisclosed, undiscussed and undocumented types of abuses and suggest a different approach to sustainably stamp out abuse of all types. This memoir deems abuse as a kind of virus that creeps into organisations the moment that the organisation fails to adopt best practices of Human Resource Management and protect everyone's human rights, especially right to do their job of providing care and support services without being abused by their service users, service users relatives or management/fellow staff members/other stakeholders.

Do not forget a hurt/hurting Carer

I have several times heard a Carer spoke very bitterly about how she was punched in her jaw by a resident and the following day she returned to work, neither the manager nor her deputy asked her how her jaw was or how she felt. More Carers narrated their own similar disappointment after hearing her. A little compassionate care or show of concern by the management to a hurt Carer does a great deal of reassuring to the Carer that she or he is not forgotten/alone or neglected and her injuries are well noted. But if your manager did not notice a punch in the jaw, would the manager be expected to notice an injury such as loss of pregnancy? That is the way Carers view it. Compassionate care is very reciprocal. Reassurance stops the Carer from taking it personally. Love and compassion are what makes a house a home. The issue of abuse in a care home is significantly related to a severe lack of love and compassion.

Celebrate every one's birthday not just residents

Staff members must remember to celebrate residents' birthdays, but their own birthdays are never celebrated at work. No staff will ever complain about the company's management, colleagues and residents not wishing him or her a happy birthday but deep down, they will notice that no one else cares. This is enough to keep that staff's mind in the direction of losing its compassion for the job and management. The residents can be spared of any blame due to their not being able to know whose birthday is due.

Confidentiality

In care homes and maybe in other workplaces, staff private folders, information and details are recklessly held. When they phone in sick, they are required to disclose why and what exactly is wrong with them to their fellow colleagues. I have seen people's filled sickness report forms hanging on notice boards in the administration office in full view of their colleagues who take handover information in the office and stay there to update daily notes and so on. Several illnesses such as staff having period pain, another had depression etc are displayed for all to see. Guess she would be further depressed if she found out that everyone knows why she rang in sick. The drawer where staff private files are stored has been usually unlocked and sometimes open to the point where staff got angry and collected his folder. It was very funny that our manager discussed confidentiality at a staff meeting bitterly warning about divulging confidential information to relatives but did not mention management and administration's own recklessness. In another care home, they installed a camera in the staff changing room located in the basement of the building.

Self-neglecting

Is it right to demand that Carers plead or beg residents to receive personal care, food or other services?

You may add to the above question, 'kneel down to beg' residents to receive personal care whether the Carer wants to or not as long as such gesture is the sort of thing that works in order to successfully give a 'self-neglecting' resident care. On the other hand, is it a form of mentally degrading a Carer or promoting the body language or subconsciously insinuating to Carers that they must succeed to Carer for everyone at all cost no matter what it takes? Take, for instance, a Carer politely explaining to a resident that it is mealtime and she has brought her food to assist her to eat. The resident understands clearly but cannot be bothered to open her mouth for the food to come in. If a resident is offered a shower or shaves and refuses if kneeling down and begging the resident had worked with other Carers, should it become a norm and be expected of other Carers to do the same even if they don't want to? Shouldn't a Carer's integrity matter?

I observed many times my colleagues beg and plead before giving assistance and then thanked residents after assisting them and I asked why did you do that? There is nothing wrong with being polite, it is indeed professional to be polite. But there is a huge difference between being polite and being timid. Reducing Carers' self-confidence to a level of timid by design is a strong blow to their self-confidence. Being timid in the sense of Carers being easily and always frightened that a resident may slap or hit or verbally, physically or sexually abuse them and the management's recognition of such acts as collateral damage and something that goes with the job.

All animals are equal, but

The management's fear or subconscious proclamation that a particular resident [or because of his or her relative] should be feared or treated better than others or given luxurious royal-like service beyond normal service does very quickly translate into various unimaginable reactions from Carers who perceive that subconscious directive.

In this care home that I worked at, a very hard-to-please resident complained about the central heating system not heating her room as much as she would have liked so an electric fan heater was given to her. But the fact that this fan heater was kept in her room for weeks and she considered it hers. But the very weird thing is that she has not used it for over a week since it was provided because in actual sense, her bedroom heating was just fine even before this fan heater was provided. One night in mid-December, one of the care home's boiler wasn't working and some bedrooms were affected but the resident with fan heater, her room wasn't affected and to my greatest astonishment, other Carers were extremely afraid and discouraged taking the fan heater from her room to give to another resident whose bedroom was extremely cold. I took the fan heater and gave it to another resident and before morning the nurse on duty told me to make sure that I return it back to this hard-to-please resident. The pressure to ensure that this resident is well pleased at the expense of others is so ridiculously huge.

In another care home I angrily questioned the act of removing a floor sensor mat from a resident who is at risk of fall to give it to another resident just because his son wanted him to have one despite that he didn't need it. His son had reported the care home to the local safeguarding team numerous times, and they were afraid of him.

All hands-on deck at rush hour

To avoid night Carers waking residents up too early in a bid to reduce the extreme morning rush hour which is a constant problem in all care homes. Get the night staff to do most of the morning cleaning for cleaners, peel potatoes cut the vegetables for the cooks. The idea is for night staff to do as much morning jobs as possible in the early hours 3 am, 4 am of each morning so that the cook and cleaners can assist with feeding and serving breakfast to allow morning Carers focus solely on getting people properly washed and dressed and avoid complaints result from rushed personal care or skipping of dental care. If any resident with mental health issues declines personal care, his or her relative should be contacted and the relative should be willing to come to the home and assist in giving reassurance and get the personal care done properly as opposed to coming to the home to blast the Carers. All hands should be on deck.

Carers against big-ego nurses

This bit here is the saddest I must add to this memoir. I once overheard a nurse telling a Carer to go to the university and study nursing and then work in a nursing home so that she will not have to assist any resident with personal care (she did use far ridiculous words which I have to not use here). This is a hint into the mindset of many nurses who work with Carers in nursing homes. These sorts of nurses assume that certain tasks are totally not theirs. I have seen this occur too many times. In one storey 26 bedding nursing home, I was working with a nurse and a Carer. The Carer and I began the bi-hourly rounds while the nurse sat in the dining room using her phone. We had a gentleman downstairs near the dining room who tries to get out of bed very often despite his being unsteady on his feet and requires urgent attention else he would fall should he attempt to stand. A sensor mat was in place to alert the team as soon as he steps on it. During the bi-hour rounds, we had to also pause several times to attend to the call bells and see the nurse still seated and texting with her phone. But when we were upstairs in the farthest corner of the building and in the middle of assisting a man with serious challenging behaviour and during this point, the gentleman downstairs got up and fell in his room. The nurse did not answer the call bell. This is one incident but I have seen it repeatedly and it appears that some nurses believe that they were at nursing homes to do the medication rounds and paperwork but will not assist the Carers even when there are serious demands and volume of their tasks increase. They often cannot be bothered to do checks by themselves and they will ask the Carers hope everyone is alright after the Carers had done the routine checks. Sometimes, they will go against the procedures and send Carers with medicines to deliver to a resident in the bedroom. I would like to request all nursing home managers to understand this issue exists and it is destroying teams and hurting compassionate care. All hands must be on deck.

Train nurses to provide care
At this nursing home, we usually have 3 Carers and a nurse working each night. The nurses only do medication and then sit down all night either updating the resident's night-time care plan or doing nothing. The directors got upset with the amount of money spent on agency Carers when a night Carer called in sick and forced the number down to 2 Carers and one nurse and the nurse must work as a Carer once night medications are done with. The nurses hated this, and they were so annoyed. They did not know how to do Carers' jobs. Things that are done as a Carer walks into a resident's bedroom before personal care like drawing window curtains, raising the bed up to prevent too much bending of the back, keeping the resident informed of each manoeuvre prior to starting it and lots of other things. The nurses did not know them. The Carers realised that the nurses are worse than the agency Carers as they do not know these things. Besides, most of the nurses are retired public sector NHS workers who still want to earn a few pounds for whatever reason(s) which means that they are too old for the physical nature of the job especially the long walks involved and the stressful nature of it. The director had to return things back to the way it was when the resignation began to increase in numbers.

Immunizations/vaccinations should be free of charge
All relevant immunisation must be provided by care homes and government for staff and free of charge basis. Immunization/vaccination is a form of personal protection from the hazards of the job hence it is an employer's responsibility. GPs still charge £15 for each dose of the Measles Mumps and

Rubella vaccination. If flu vaccine is provided free of charge, then other work-related vaccines should be free.

NHS must stop extortion of Carers

According to the evening standard online news on 27th December 2017, "

NHS hospitals make a record £174m from car parking...

Patients, visitors, and staff paid a mammoth total of £174,526,970 in parking charges in 2016/17, up to six per cent the year before.

Data collected by the Press Association also revealed hospital trusts raked in £947,568 in parking fines from patients, visitors, and staff.

"staff include Carers who are on low income. Carers on near minimum wage income pay the exact same amount as surgeons and directors to park their little car and begin their shift on time. The worst is the local council institute residents-with-permit only parking in all surrounding streets of the hospital so Carers cannot even Park anywhere near the hospital. This is daylight extortion and destruction of compassion in care. It should be stopped immediately.

Carers' taxi expenses especially Christmas and other bank holidays should be deducted from the gross income before tax is deducted and should be done by the payroll who must inform Carers to submit such fare receipts.

I wrote this piece in early 2018 and during the 2020 coronavirus epidemic, Carers became the most needed manpower called, 'key workers' and the Health Secretary wrote the Carers a letter promising free parking. Why charge them in the first place? Sadly, as soon as Coronavirus lockdown began to ease, there were Newspaper reports that government want to re-introduce the parking fees.

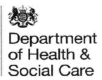

Department
of Health &
Social Care

28 March 2020

To my brilliant colleagues in social care,

The last few weeks have been difficult for all of us. I am acutely conscious that you, along with colleagues across the health and social care system, are on the front line caring for and supporting people in incredibly challenging circumstances. Many of the people you care for will be in groups that are at higher risk from Covid-19 and I know that you will have naturally felt concerned for them. At the same time, you will have been grappling with the same issues we all face: how we can best keep ourselves and our loved ones healthy, juggling our own personal caring responsibilities, and looking out for our friends, our neighbours and communities.

My main message to you is simple: thank you.

Thank you for going the extra mile to make sure the people who rely on you are supported. Thank you in advance for the difficult decisions you will have to make that will keep as many people as possible safe. Thank you for taking on extra shifts to cover for those who need to isolate or have their own caring responsibilities. Thank you for doing the right thing by isolating if you or somebody you live with has symptoms. Thank you for everything you are doing this week, next week and in the months to come.

We face more difficult times ahead and I know you will have been personally impacted by the measures we have had to take to reduce the spread of Covid-19. Whilst many people are now staying at home, I know that is not an option for most of you as your work, caring for others, cannot be done from home. We will do all we can to make your lives easier during this period, including, for example, making parking on council owned on-street spaces and car parks free for those who work in social care.

The Government is releasing advice and information updates daily and we are working round the clock to make sure you and your employer have the information, equipment and resources you need. For those of you that use Twitter, please follow the Department for Health and Social Care (@DHSCgovuk) for the latest information. We will also make it available through other channels. I also want to reiterate what the Chancellor has said: we are committed to doing whatever is needed; that promise applies just as much to social care as it does for the NHS.

Thank you again for everything you do.

Yours ever,

MATT HANCOCK

113

End unpaid 'trial/voluntary Shifts'

It is very sad that this exploitation is legally happening in the era. I have had my fair share and I dealt with it well. I arrived at the interview when the manager told me that they had a policy of giving me the opportunity to see if I like the job or not and that is the voluntary shift that I must do. I got home after the interview and gave it a thought. I am a very experienced Carer and I know what the job requires so why force me to volunteer? I asked myself. I sent her an email afterwards, see my email and her (manager) response below.

"Dear - - -
I am considerably keen to work at - - -House. I would be delighted to provide further information if required, undergo full induction, work shadowing and be on probation for up to 6 months or more within which you can freely dismiss me even after my first shift if I performed poorly. However, as a matter of personal principle, I humbly regret to inform you that I will not be available for 23rd April's voluntary half shift for you to check whether or not your current employees would like me before you decide to employ me. I am very interested to start as soon as I have been offered the job. If this is against your company's policy or procedure, I would totally understand. Thanks very much for the opportunity. Kindest   Regards"

Her   reply

**"Good   Morning   Chuck,
I can start your training immediately in which case.
The voluntary shift is not a compulsory feature of our**

recruitment process, rather one that we find works for us as a team. You will be on a one month trial period, whereby we can discuss contracting at the end of this month. Kind Regards

KF
Registered Manager"

When I finally started working, my colleagues asked why I did not do the voluntary shift and I said I cannot be forced to volunteer. They were surprised that I didn't do it and said to me that they didn't know that the 'voluntary' shift wasn't compulsory the way it was presented to them at interview and one lady said she felt that if she did not do the unpaid shift, she would not have been employed.

Deliberately planned no room for handover
CQC and local safeguarding authorities once again failed to question why the staff will have finished their shift (e.g. 8:00am) at the same time the new incoming team commenced their shift at the exact same time (8:00am). It is either there's no handover or that staff are forced to work longer than their finished work time without any pay or staff are forced to arrive and start working early without pay before they are due to start.

Other form of extortion
Rip-off of Carers (late timesheet submission deduction and losing untaken annual leave) should be considered fraud.
There is a care agency in Leicester that deducts money from their Carers should they submit their current week timesheet (invoice) late (afternoon time next week Monday). Is it lawful, moral and right to do that? The only punishment for late submission of

timesheets should be late processing and payment. It is very ridiculous that some care recruitment agencies steal from Carers in the so-called late timesheet submission fee. This fee is charged by agencies that supply temporary staff to care homes, therefore Some care home managers may assume it does not concern them but hurting a Carer kills compassionate care and a Carer without compassion renders any qualifications or training absolutely useless. That is how it concerns you.

No Carer should lose untaken holidays since there are numerous rules preventing them from taking their holidays when they want, a good example of such rules include; no two day or night Carers can take their annual leave at the same time and no annual leave will be approved in the month of December up to the first week of January of the following year. One Carer must wait until the other has returned and must not take a holiday between December and the first week of January. This begins to look like the management are deliberately finding ways to fraudulently make the Carers lose some of their annual leave allowance which the management has already stipulated that they will not be paid if it is not taken. On 29th December, I applied for annual leave for 30th January carefully giving one-month notice as required. I got the following reply from the management, "Your Holiday request for 30/01/2020 has been declined due to the rota already been done" and when I phoned for clarification, I argued that rota being already done in ahead should not be a reason since I adhered to the one month notice period. To this I was told that the management can also disapprove of any annual leave if there is no staff to cover the shifts.

Annual leave should be accrued by both permanent, part-time and Bank staff and all accrued annual leave by Carers both permanent, part-time and Bank staff should be paid to the Carer even when the annual leave was not taken by the time the yearly cycle ends.

Being on low income means either taking government benefits to supplement the income or working longer hours and more shifts per week at same job or adding a second job to earn more income. It goes up to the extent of Carers accepting holiday pay but working during their annual leave either for the employer or elsewhere. It is not greed; it is rather attempting to meet their needs.

Lateness to work wage deductions

Generally, it seems to me that managers and other top-level decision makers are oblivious to the logistical needs of their employees and this manifests in various policies which they implement. They are also oblivious to the fact that shortage of Carers means that they cannot get enough Carers from their immediate community and must employ Carers from little distance and also the fact that Carers earn 'peanuts' so can't afford to buy, insure and maintain a vehicle for work purposes. They also do not realise that It is normal human instinct for any worker who arrives late to work to hurry up, hang the coat and join the rest of the team and that is exactly what the Carers I have observed did despite what the company's lateness punishment policy states.

This deduction involves summary deduction of Carer's time as punishment for lateness. In this care home I was working, any Carer who arrives to work late by 1 minute will forfeit 15 minutes of paid time. This has happened to many Carers and when it happened to me.

Every Saturday when my local football team Leicester FC plays their home match, there will be increased traffic along the route that I will be taking to work. But on this evening, the chairman of Leicester FC died right there in the stadium car park after the football match when his helicopter crashed and there were fire service and police. When I received my payslip, I asked for an explanation and got a response through the phone as well as through my email, "As discussed on the telephone your hours paid is correct, deduction due to lateness on 2 days".

These deductions will not stop traffic from holding a Carer up preventing the Carer from arriving early next time. This punishment is foolish and a deliberate dent and spat at whatever compassionate care that exists. Carers are already in the lowest paid category, why would lowering pay any further by lateness deductions be helping to boost morale? This is simply a case of a well-paid manager who can afford to get a reliable vehicle, who works sort of 9 to 5 hours so arrives to work after the sun is out and leaves before the sun sets hence knew nothing about odd hours and public transport reliability, such a person making policies that affect people on lowest income. For such a manager who is on over £30,000 per year may need this cruel policy magnifying for the manager to see that making a Carer work for 14 minutes unpaid because the Carer was 1 minute late is same as making a Carer work for 14 hours unpaid because the Carer was 1 hour late.

Perpetual lateness should attract disciplinary warning but Carers who rely solely on public transport are likely to arrive late once or twice each month. The Carer may also arrive home late from work due to traffic. While being late by one minute may rationally or logically attract a one-minute deduction from the Carer's wage if there must be a deduction for absent time in a tit-for-tat sort of environment, going beyond tit-for-tat or eye for an eye to deduct 15:1 ratio is absurd. There are instruments called calculators as well as online websites and payroll computer applications which can help any office administrator work out the monetary worth of a minute rather than summary deduction. There are also times when due to huge demands or other factors the Carers do not leave the work premises by the end of their shift, these extra times are not worked out with the same principle of lateness wage deductions. If so, then if a Carer leaves a minute later than supposed to, then 15 minutes should be added to the Carer's total hours. Ask yourself, why would any Carer spend a minute more than paid for at this care home that is implementing this policy? It takes away any compassionate care that exists. One evening in the middle of October, I turned up to the central bus station and waited for the bus to work and none turned up. When I realised that the next bus would mean I will be almost an hour late, I decided to cancel going to work entirely. I just cannot start to imagine how much they will deduct from my wage for being nearly an hour late and I will need a taxi to get back in the morning, so it was totally worthless. They should get the agency staff to cover since they cannot tolerate their staff being late not even once and not even if it was for an unforeseeable circumstance. I did tell them my plumbing had packed up and my house was flooded, and I took the next bus to go back home. On my way they rang begging me to go even in the middle of the night after a plumber has been but did not say anything about the cost of midnight taxi but guess that's pending if I even want to go. How pathetic is the fact that the motivation was terribly low? No such thing as solidarity.

When clocks go hour forward
It is unspeakable to find out that various care homes do not pay their night Carers the extra hour that they will be working when clocks go an hour forward usually in October of every year. This should be condemned by the strongest of terms.

The timetable should be designed to prevent night staff getting caught up in the morning rush hour traffic. They have been awake all night and deserve to get home safely and quickly to get some sleep. The shift pattern should be offered by the management to the prerogative of the Carers to either accept or reject finishing early enough before the rush hour begins. In Leicester for instance, if the night shift finishes at 7:30am, one can get home before rush hour kicks off because the children and families start school run around 7:50am onwards.

Sunday mornings offer (reduce taxi use)
Some night Carers who rely on public transport may have to wait until 09:00am after finishing their shift at 08:00am for the public buses to start running or go home on a taxi which usually costs around 10% of whatever they earned that night. If the management could offer them a better alternative such as staying a little longer but recognise the fact that they will be very tired so not like try get their money worth of labour off any Carer who agrees to stay in for the little longer, Carers who are affected may accept this alternative. It is indeed in your best interest because many Carers might just call in sick rather than lose over 10% of already taxed income to taxi fare. That is exactly how it works.

Pay Carers for being on call
Please read the following text:
"The Christmas rota is almost finished and will be put up shortly so that you can see what shifts you have been allocated.
I still need, however, someone to be on-call on Christmas Day.
On-call staff are paid on Christmas Eve, Christmas Day and Boxing Day night (£25) whether you get called in or not.
Any volunteers?"

The only issue with this is that if the company recognises the need to compensate Carers who were put on-call all night but did not get called in, why compensate only Christmas and Boxing but won't compensate on non-season periods? The employment laws are still far from protecting employees (Carers) from different sorts of ridiculous ways that they are being short-changed by their employers. I have added this bit to the memoir because to achieve a greater level of compassionate care, then all these unfair practices must cease to exist.

Wage underpayment problems

I preferred to discuss underpayment because all the payroll never made any overpayment error in all cases, it was always an underpayment. It starts from induction day and happens because Carers often get their key fobs and begin to use it to sign in and out from their next shift after the induction shift and for this reason, their induction shift is never paid leading up to their first underpayment.

There should be a system of issuing payslips in a few working days before payday. Alternatively, Carers should be informed how many hours they will be paid and how this affects their total to-be-paid hours was calculated before payday so that any error can be rectified in time and the right amount is paid in that month. This is because most companies argue that any underpayment can only be paid in the next pay period which is in a month's time.

Zero-Hour Contracts and Recruitment agency staffs

Poor support for new and agency Carers

An agency Carer covering a shift, Doing the hot drinks, for instance, does not know the residents, who has sugar, who can swallow biscuits, needs thickened fluid. If someone chokes and dies, that agency Carer may be looking at defending self against manslaughter charges. As simple as that. Every resident has a big folder containing pages of that resident's care plan. It will take several weeks for a new Carer to read these Carers to know each resident. Agency Carers do not have the time or opportunity to read this care plan folder, yet they are expected to care for the residents. The best alternative way is to keep asking teammates but try asking stressed busy teammates continuously and you find it is easier to just risk it than getting on their frustrated nerves. They are tired and just cannot entertain constantly asking them questions after questions. If an agency Carer is about serving 40 cups of tea then ask 40 times if each individual need thickened tea or if the resident can chew and swallow biscuits safely or isn't diabetic so can have sugar or drinks with a special beaker, not teacup or etc.

Zero hours contracts and suspensions

I know an agency Carer working at a council-owned home on behalf of a recruitment agency. One day an allegation was made that required the manager to suspend all Carers who were on that early shift pending the outcome of an investigation. The investigation took a month. Permanent council employees who were part of the suspension were paid as normal. The agency Carers were not. After one month, they were all cleared of any wrongdoing, but no compensation was paid and on return to their recruitment company, we are told that since they have been off work for over a month, they need to re-register. And their pay which increases after six months will return to minimum wage. This is true and factual. Carers on zero-hour contracts get punished for no wrongdoing.

Unsocial Hours Pay
This is one of the issues the government should intervene to advocate that night staff get better rates as well as Christmas and New year and bank holidays. Carers union may seem far from reality but individual striking and loss of compassion for the job and for residents in Carers' care are growing seriously. Pay transport bonuses for a taxi on holidays. The problem of transportation during Bank Holiday, Xmas and New Year and similar times like striking transport workers should not be the sole burden of employees.

Too weak, neglected and undermined to speak
The first day I went to work in this country in early 2011, the food processing factory had these speakers tuned on FM radio which played the lazy song by Bruno Mars over and over. The lyrics which included, "today I don't feel like doing anything. I just wanna lay in my bed" was louder and louder. This song was a hit track, but this is also the song which Britain's radio stations played over and over for a working man during working hours on a working day. The reaction was either no one else noticed or just like me whoever noticed could not speak up. Why didn't any of the workers say something since it is unimaginable that they were enjoying the music which was competing with sounds of our machines over which one can damage our ears first? Workers on the lowest level of the system rarely speak up. They are just too tired, weak or neglected to say something. In the UK, doctors

and nurses do go on strike to persuade the government and other stakeholders to improve the safety of patients, pay and general work welfare. The only group of workers who are treated far worse than the doctors and nurses but who have never been on strike are the Carers. This is dangerous because it leads to burying animosity instead of addressing it and this happens very subconsciously on a very large scale across the length and breadth of the country.

End Forced Labour

Forced labour existing in Care Homes

Care homes do not like to use emergency care staff from a recruitment agency due to the high fees they charge. Some care homes offer their permanent or bank/relief staff higher rates of pay to tempt them to pick up an extra shift or emergency shifts that may be required to be covered when it's allocated staff phone in sick a few hours before commencement. I have no problem with that. But there are other care homes who compel their staff to pick up those emergency shifts. They do it by allocating a staff each day to be on standby (on call) and be ready to come to work should someone phone sick. This 'on call' shift is certainly not part of the staff's contracted weekly or monthly hours. It is, in other words, forcing the staff to work extra hours or to anticipate and prepare to do so. This makes it forced labour whether it is written on the contract or not considering that in case of human trafficking, both the trafficker and the victim usually have binding agreements beforehand but nonetheless it is still human trafficking. Football teams do pay all players whether on reserve bench or in field playing. Therefore, if you want someone to be on reserve (on-call or standby) on a contract basis, you must pay the staff as if the staff worked on that particular day and it must be included in weekly hours and put in contract as hours worked. This wicked act kills compassionate care because the management has through its intimidation and contractual manipulation forced its Carer to come to work when the Carer did not want or apply to work and to work beyond the weekly hours that the Carer agreed to work. It is forced labour.

Bank holiday forced workers

Carers must go to work on Christmas and new year and a public holiday for no extra pay. They will not be allowed to take a holiday in December. They are not allowed to. It is true the residents' needs must be met but the government must indicate the red line. For instance, the law could be amended to reserve two of either Christmas, New Year or Easter day/night for each Carer. So, if a Carer works on Christmas then that Carer must be allowed to spend the new year with family and not be forced to work on the new year. The Carers are mostly not paid any extra for these bank holidays and they must pay for a taxi to go to work and return home because the buses do not run on bank holidays. There is a developing trend where December sees lots of resignations and January sees lots of job applications.

Easter, Christmas, New Year and school holiday rota

Christmas Rotas

Please tick next to the box you would like to work over the Christmas period full time staff you need to work the equivalent of 2 full days, 1 full day and 2 ½ days or 4 ½ days. This is not the finishing rota!! If I cannot fill it with EVERYONES help then I will have no choice but to revert back to normal rota!!

Thanks

Kym

Name :

Christmas Day 8am-2pm	Boxing Day 8am-2pm	New Year's Eve 8am-2pm	New Year's Day 8am-2pm
2pm-8pm	2pm-8pm	2pm-8pm	2pm-8pm

Christmas Day 6am-12pm	Boxing Day 6am-12pm	New Year's Eve 6am-12pm	New Year's Day 6am-12pm
12pm-6pm	12pm-6pm	12pm-6pm	12pm-6pm

Christmas Day 8pm-8am	Boxing Day 8pm-8am	New Year's Eve 8pm-8am	New Year's Day 8pm-8am

This is the most important rota for all care homes, and it is very important that the manager looks at the rota before it is published/posted on the notice board to ensure rational and fairness. Start by ensuring the two core days/nights (Christmas, new year and Easter days and nights) are shared equally among staff. Then equally share the peripherals (Christmas eve, new year eve, boxing day, Good Friday, Easter Monday) days/nights making sure everyone gets one core and one peripheral day/night according to the shift pattern they do. If possible, offer them their chosen picks, for instance, if staff want to work on Christmas rather than a new year, then let the staff have it if you can. No staff must be allowed to take holiday on these holiday dates. All staff who do not rely on public buses to travel to work, as well as those who do not celebrate Christmas and Easter, may be asked to volunteer using any suitable motivation but never compel them to or use threats. Furthermore, holiday booking for children holiday periods as well as mid-term break weeks should be shared among all applicants rather than on a first come first served basis. staff who do not have children may be encouraged to book non-children holiday weeks for their annual leave and use any suitable motivation but never compel them to or use threats.

Heatwaves

Carers working under extreme temperatures

In cold temperatures, care homes often raise heater temperature to meet the needs of residents. This is good because residents are mostly inactive sitting down for the most part of the day. On the other hand, Carers are climbing up and down the stairs, running from one corner of the home to the other and wearing a uniform which is usually thick, then when the home temperature is increased their own body temperature goes sky high. In the night, the care home windows must be closed for security reasons, this makes it impossible for fresh air to get into the care home at that time. This lack of ventilation is furthermore heightened in grade two listed Victoria era buildings being used for care home purpose now since in these buildings the windows do not open at all some of its hinges will be rusted. It's bad for the environment as by the end of the day when the dining room and lounges will be cleaned, you see dead bees and wasps over a hundred of them that flew into the building and die since they won't find a way out. Over a hundred of them every day.

This temperature issue has led to a miscarriage of pregnancies, collapse, exhaustion and so on and all remain unreported. Right now, I challenge anyone to do this research and you will see that Carers have a higher than average rate of pregnancy miscarriages in the UK. The fact that more kindness and stronger demand for justice is shown in animal case such as this April 2019 The Independent news report that, "Two men have been arrested after a horse, which is believed to be pregnant, collapsed on a main street in Cardiff city centre on the hottest day of the year so far....on suspicion of causing unnecessary suffering to a protected animal". Someone from the sanctuary where the horse was taken after it managed to stand up, said the horse was "exhausted and suffering from heatstroke which could have been fatal." A similar thing happens regularly in care homes to human beings.

There must be a way to meet the needs of residents and meet the Carers' needs. Allow them to wear a thin uniform or mufti to work in such times, allow 10 minutes outdoors or air-conditioned room break after every 2 hours. Instead of the usual trousers, knee-length chinos short of your organisation colour can do.

On July 22nd, 2019, I received a text message from management, **"Until Sunday staff relaxed uniform for the week. Sandals must have a back for your safety. Vest tops shorts skirts etc. Pls wear aprons to protect ur personal clothing during every intervention.   Thanks"**.

The first time ever that I received this sort of message and I have been working in the industry since 2013. I received the message a long time after I had written this paragraph and subsequent paragraphs relating to heatwave and I was surprised but glad that things are improving. However, it requires a national or nationwide sort of change which only the CQC and/or health and safety executive can affect because relaxing uniform policy in one care home is good but until it is done in every care home then it is not enough.

Record Highs

Furthermore, A lot of buildings in the UK are designed to trap heat. With climate change, we have been seeing record-breaking summer heat temperatures. The issue is that the entire care is designed to ensure the welfare of residents but at the extreme expense of the Carers. The management offices have air conditioning systems to cool their offices down. However, Carers who are always on their feet walking down and up the corridors and due to this physical nature, their body temperature goes way higher than already extreme inside the building temperature in already extreme national temperature. Some Carers will lose their pregnancy and they will not take it any further than crying in their lonely time. Most managers have heard about a Carer or more losing pregnancy in the summer period and I can write this because it is happening again and again. The rule that only one Carer can take annual leave at any time means that they will not be able to take time off work and must work under this extreme temperature and pressure. The high temperature often leads to emergency fire exit doors left wide open by Carers and in few cases by residents in order to let in some fresh air which rarely comes in because UK buildings are designed for cold weathers to trap heat and prevent cold air coming into the building from outside. This has in numerous times led to missing person situations as some residents with dementia may leave the property without anyone noticing. The solution is simple and easy, and it is called an air conditioning system in all corridors and lounges and residents' rooms. If the temperature degrees keep to the thirties and forties year by year, then the climate change issues are not going away any sooner and the air conditioning system should be prioritised just as the gas central heating system has been. Maybe the air conditioning system can be powered by solar panels to take advantage of the long sunshine and turn it into useful cooling energy at a cheaper cost.

Review of NHS guidelines a heatwave in 2019

In May 2019, the Public Health England, Department of Health and Social Care, and NHS England released documents, "Heatwave Plan for England" and "heatwave SUPPORTING VULNERABLE PEOPLE
BEFORE AND DURING A HEATWAVE

Advice for care home managers and staff" respectively. I will review only the one that was sent to the care home where I worked which is the NHS version titled, "Heatwave Supporting Vulnerable People Before and During a Heatwave Advice for care home managers and staff"

This good document unfortunately focused on the protection of residents only and didn't recognise that during the same heatwave, Carers who are actively walking and running from one corner of the building to the other, climbing stairs and absorbing stress some of whom are pregnant could at that particular point in time be also classed as vulnerable people. For instance, an advice like this one on page six, "Check that residents have light, loose-fitting cotton clothing" is an obvious indicator of the callousness I'm talking about in this memoir since the same advice could have been worded like this, "Check that staff, as well as residents, have light, loose-fitting cotton clothing" while highlighting need to suspend or relax any adverse uniform policy for the duration of the heatwave.

The documents also lacked the following.

It did not advise any safeguarding measures for Carers including pregnant Carers who would also be working during the heatwave. It didn't discuss the major issues during heatwave which includes the fact that care homes including modern purpose built and another grade two listed buildings have extremely intricate heating/temperature adjustment switches and only a trained maintenance personnel can adjust it and fact that temperature can go from 2 degrees at midnight and early morning up to 20 degrees in the afternoon and late afternoon and stays around that region until it starts to cool down again when sunsets and there's no maintenance personnel to adjust the heating accordingly. The documents did mention checking the temperature of the home at least four times each day but never mentioned that Carers should be trained to adjust or turn off the heating and how to turn it back on when necessary. The heater remains at full blast during some heat waves because the temperature fluctuates too cold in the night, too hot in the day and no one (Carer) knows how to control it and the maintenance personnel may have gone home or works only a few days a week. Some care homes do not have any maintenance personnel or are on holiday or work part-time like twice each week as I already wrote. Today is the 25th of July 2019, the UK has "recorded its second hottest day ever, with temperatures reaching 38.1C" and hottest July day ever in recorded history of as reported by BBC News and guess what, I started a night shift yesterday 24th July and as I sat next to a gas central heating in the conservatory about 22:30, I realised that the heating was on. The heating was also not turned off by the time I returned for another night shift on the evening of the 25th of July. Despite all the warnings to push fluid, give residents light clothing etc. I do not know how to turn off the entire central heating since this is a completely complex system different from one in my house. Some of the heating panels were off while others were on. That is why it is a completely complicated system. The heat was unbearable, and the shift was hard one. The next morning (26th of July 2019) when day Carers arrived, I spoke to the senior (team leader) Carer to ensure that the heating were turned off and she said that they knew about it already but the maintenance man had gone on holiday to Poland and no one else knows how to do it. This is exactly what the makers of this document should be campaigning for.

I also have one more issue, I received this text message, "Good morning everyone just to let you all know that ALL RESIDENTS ARE ON FLUID CHART UNTILL SUNDAY PLEASE PUSH FLUIDS AS MUCH AS POSSIBLE

Thanks"

I wish it was worded differently to include Carers. It could have said All residents are on a fluid chart and so on but includes that all Carers and other staff must take a few minutes of every hour to have a cold refreshing drink. A shower room with some towels may also be reserved specifically for Carers to shower whenever they felt unbearably hot.

The documents also failed to discuss the fire risk in the boiler room which in most care homes is where laundry equipment is kept and laundry is done and this room is hot, dry, dusty and just needs only a spark to trigger a fire. The documents are so shallow that one can see that the creators have never worked in any old people's care home as front-line care staff. There is evidence of deep thought into creating this document, as a matter of fact, the creator in page 9, suggested adjustments to the working arrangement that may include recalling Carers who are on holiday and making changes to rotas but none of such thought went into the welfare of the staff during the heatwave.

The most foolish part of this was that one of the few times the report mentioned 'staff' was referring to asking staff who are on their annual leave holiday to cut it and return to work. Totally ignored the fact that by law, a Carer/staff cannot be forced, rather can only agree to do so out of compassion but ask yourself, why would any of such Carer cut short their holiday when the work environment is dreadful with zero care/attention to staff wellbeing during the heatwave. Dehydration as an issue is discussed completely on part of the residents and not a single thought is spared to consider the Carers. Asking for installation of an air conditioning system in all care homes for these heat waves may be asking too much.

Allocate staff to close bedroom Windows

In many care homes, especially during the winter months, bedroom windows are usually open from the morning when the Carers open them to let in some fresh air to the point when residents go to bed. This means that residents go into very cold rooms and risk pneumonia and that is beside the energy Wastage in terms of a higher cost of heating the premises. No one cares it seems but, this happens because no one bothers to allocate it to staff with most managers leaving the building around 5pm and they do not know first-hand what goes on after that time.

Coronavirus

Complacent handling of Coronavirus

Coronavirus epidemic was a disaster. To understand why, you need to rule out why not. Developing a suitable strategy was not the issue since the UK has handled other viral infections such as HIV. Taking HIV for instance, all adverts in the billboard in UK focussed on testing and condom while in other countries it also included being faithful to one sexual partner. Applying these key 'coherent actions' of dealing with HIV virus to Coronavirus, Testing remains testing while Condom becomes Face covering and being faithful to one partner becomes stopping use of agency carers or regulating their use to working in one care home only. Forget about isolation or lockdown, these are necessary coherent actions but they are post-infection actions in other words, they are actions that are taken after the virus had spread and they are extremely ineffective as well as economically expensive which meant that they are not sustainable.

The virus tore through the UK in March and April while Carers first got tested in my first job in first week of June 2020. Similarly, use of face covering in public transport was mandated in June 2020 and later, use of face covering in shops was to be enforced in July. These two coherent actions got to me as an individual in June 2020 whereas the virus infection spiked in March 2020 to an uncontrollable level. Face covering could have been made a law from February 2020 at zero cost. Government lied that they did not introduce mandatory use of face masks to prevent it running out for the NHS key workers at the fore front of fighting the virus in hospitals. This is a lie since a mere folded double handkerchief with rubber band could have been a good face covering.

The stage-by-stage strategy was the biggest failure. The Corona virus required a simultaneous guidance policy and coherent actions. The stage one (containment), two (delay) and three (research) should have been implemented at the same time. The stage one (containment) failed because of failure to do testing and failure to mandate face covering. The research stage can be criticised since everyone knew about the virus as far back as November 2019 while it was ravaging Chinese Wuhan county.

I mentioned the 'condom' and 'being faithful to one partner' as key coherent action in HIV control strategy, In care homes, use of agency Carers who worked in many care homes was the biggest risk factor coupled with residents that are discharged from hospital without being tested. The earlier factor (agency carers) was never regulated throughout the pandemic which caused the care home situation to worsen while the testing of residents leaving hospitals gradually increased.

Corona virus at my second job

When the coronavirus epidemic got to the UK, I had already slowed down with writing this memoir and I got other things keeping me busy such as a wife and a pregnant one for that matter. Anyway, I watched things I wrote in this Memoir beginning with the neglect of the government to add care home coronavirus deaths to the national data. I also noticed that the government suddenly gave Carers and NHS workers free parking.

I resigned my second job because on 19th April 2020, there were very strong suspicions that the virus may have made its way to our care home and a doctor had written Covid-19 on a resident's death certificate despite her not getting tested and having a history of pneumonia. The public health England took samples from two residents who were coughing nonstop. Residents were restricted to staying in respective rooms. That same night, we arrived at work worried and at handover, a day Carer came to deliver the message from the administrator/secretary/clerk whose authority surpassed the nurses and Carers to show you the extent of the neglect the instruction she gave was that only two Carers out of three should get the face mask. I was very angry because if Covid-19 is in the premises then it may have silently spread, and I cannot work with any resident at all without a face mask. I was responsible for residents who needed a lone Carer which the category that the resident who was coughing fell into. She was asleep through the night after my colleague assisted her to bed earlier, so I made only one contact with her in the morning when I assisted her to go to her toilet. Luckily, the nurse defied the instruction and gave me a face mask which I wore. I also folded a plastic apron and wrapped over my face mask to double my protection. The resident was coughing very severely at the time. I was scared. I told the nurse when I got out of her room that I did not feel safe at all. Later in the evening I got a call from a colleague that she was tested positive for coronavirus.

My reasons for deciding against returning to work are:

A. They gave us cheap ripping gloves

B. They refused to give me face mask

C. I have a pregnant wife

D. I have two jobs. In fact, this job is my second 2 nights per week. My first job 3/4 nights per week is OK for me

E. Will I die for this country that never showed me love?

F. No death on duty benefits or insurance

I was due to return to work at my second job on the 23rd and 24th April 2020 but after telling my wife, she would not let me return to work. I was angry too, so I rang in sick while I picked up extra shifts at my first job. The next week I rang in sick again with vomiting. I must ring in sick (tell lies) until I get my last wage on 30th April or else, they will seize my hard-earned money and claim that it was used to cover my shifts. I have already made up my mind to not return after they showed absolute lack of care for their staff and did not understand the seriousness of the situation. The nurses in hospital wear adequate gloves, face/eye shield, very best quality face masks, overall apron made with good quality materials and get covered by death on service scheme. In fact, there is a move to get the insurance cover for their relatives as well. While I look at myself being given a low-quality face mask out of a nurse's defiance on 19th April. What will I be thinking if I catch the virus and pass it on to my pregnant wife?

Staff Uniforms and PPE

Nurse-like Uniforms

Shall I tell you a story? There was a time when my mum travelled with me and my siblings leaving my dad and aunt in the house. My aunt was studying nursing at a nearby University of Nigeria Teaching Hospital. My dad told us a story on our return how he had to pick my aunt from medical school to go to the local village market and do some fresh grocery shopping. She was very adamant that she must get home first before they proceed to the local market for shopping. My dad asked why since he himself had only just finished from work and rather get the shopping over with and then go home to relax and she replied she needs to change her school of nursing uniform because she doesn't want the local traders calling her 'nurse check out my products and offers' in other words, she did not want to be tagged nurse. I remember this story because you can see a young lady willing to become a nurse but not proud of the nursing uniform. This exact thing is happening today. Uniforms put young people off. Especially young men. Teenage boys rather work in warehouses than to become Carers due to reasons including mandatory uniform. The uniform put people off period. I need you to understand what I mean by uniform, it's not wearing similar coloured clothes, It is those shirts designed to look like a male nurse with stripes, numerous pockets, and even has a shoulder badge in some cases as if designed to stick a Corp rank onto. Just a simple casual high street shirt or polo shirt should be a good option and for infection control, they can wear a tabard or an apron in some cases when doing personal care. The casual shirt or polo with the tabard is far better than the nurse-like uniforms. Tabard is like an apron which can be removed or washed at the workplace daily, so it is better than uniform it stays in the workplace permanently. It is unimaginable to be expecting a young man or teenager to be walking in the streets wearing a nursing uniform. It is not cool. Talking about coolness, the 'nurse uniform' is very uncomfortable to wear in the hot summer of June and July with its 65% polyester materials which itches and causes discomfort and makes me wear an inner t-shirt to prevent the itchy feeling of polyester which will not happen if I am wearing cotton or wool materials of chinos trousers (98% cotton and 2% spandex) and polo shirts (100% cotton). The spandex makes it flexible. Managers do not wear nurses' uniform, so they have no clue what it really feels like to wear one. Such a choice is not appealing to me or to younger people. When you have older people in management who do not wear uniform making fashion-related decisions for a young dominated staff team then it is likely to be disliked or unattractive. Some young managers have moved on from the nurse-like uniforms to polo shirts, this move is commendable. Polo shirts are flexible, breathable far better than nurse-like uniforms.

Uniforms are PPE

Carers should be provided uniforms for free just like other personal protective equipment. What care homes do is strike buy one get one free deal from tailors and then lie to Carers that they should buy one and the company buy another one for them but they all know the truth and companies should stop doing it. Besides, if a Carer buys his own uniform, he has the right to wear it to his second job if he has another job and it risks infection transmission as contaminants in the uniform can spread from one care home to the other but if the uniform is provided for free and all care homes provide uniforms, then the Carer would not need to wear the same uniform to various care homes. If a Carer is wearing another care home uniform with the badge visibly displayed, then sooner or later a senior or manager may notice the badge and consider providing the Carer with his or her own uniform.

The cost of a Carer's uniform should be deducted before tax is deducted by the care home's account department since it is a core work/business related expenditure.

Carers must not go home with their work uniforms

In the food manufacturing industry or companies, the production field staff are not allowed to go home with their work uniforms and boots. They walk into the dressing room, put on their uniforms (laboratory coat) and boots, then wash & sanitise their hands, wear a hair net and then go inside the production hall and when going out, they remove the laboratory coat into a wash basket and wash the boots then hang it up. Then go home. They do not own the boots or uniforms. They do not do its washing and ironing; they do not leave with them. The fact that Carers leave with work clothes is a danger to the public.

Uniforms are extremely contagious PPE and must be considered contaminated until they are decontaminated. Uniforms that have been used but have not been decontaminated should be bagged with red bags, placed in laundry rooms for washing and must not be allowed to leave the premises until decontaminated as a public health safety measure. Uniforms should be washed, ironed and placed in each Carer's locker so that the Carer wears it on arrival to start a shift and removes it after his or her shift. This is the procedure in salad processing food factories to safeguard contamination and should be adopted in care homes. Imagine the real-life situation when our care home was in a lockdown state due to a diarrhoea outbreak, some Carers who have children reported that their children came up with the same health issue (diarrhoea) that is ongoing in our care homes before the lockdown was over.

Like-colour uniforms for washing sake

Every Carer understands the need to wash the uniform as soon as he gets home. But when you must wear black trousers and a sky-blue tunic shirt, you will realise that overtime, the trousers' black colour is turning the tunic dark in some parts. This questions the thought that goes into selecting uniforms. They do not expect that you wash them, separately do they? Besides the uniform is going straight to the washing machine because I am avoiding it making any contact with my home until it is washed and disinfected so where will I keep the top while I wash the trousers?

It is very important for me to not mix light and dark colours; the dark coloured bottom half must wait for the next loading but then keeping it in the house while it waits risks contaminating the house. It shows how little the thought that goes into this sort of planning before managers decide uniforms. Please let uniforms be either bright coloured top and bottom or dark coloured top and bottom. Considering that I have already suggested thicker trousers such as jeans, corduroy or chinos which Carers will wear both at work and on their way to work or home especially Carers who use public transport. It is also important to note that some jeans' colours do not withstand regular washing. Since work clothes are washed almost daily, management should choose a colour that will not show signs of regular washing such as those nearer to white like grey or cream. This takes away the choice of either buying jeans on a regular basis or wearing heavily washed ones.

There should be a flexible uniform policy that changes with the weather. A thin plain short or trousers in the summer and thick jeans or chinos in the colder seasons for instance.

Pyjamas day for children in need

On children in need, our manager asked us to come to work in our pyjamas rather than our uniforms to highlight & raise funds for children in need. I was the only staff who refused to abide. I told them that due to the nature of work we do, I would never use my pyjamas to do the work and if I must then I must discard my pyjamas afterwards because I will not wear it in my bed ever again. Discarding clothes which are still in good condition is a despicable act that I will not consider the environment-friendly act. Therefore, I refused to participate. This shows how little thought that was put into the planning.

Anti-Jeans/Denim policy (plain trousers only)

Most care homes have an anti-jeans policy. This policy is totally wrong because jeans are very essential clothing in the wintertime. For any Carer who walks to work or must wait long to/from a bus stop before/after work in the winter season when the temperature drops to near freezing, the Carer would tell you that a plain trouser is not suitable clothing for such weather. I once tried wearing long-John inner thermal clothing inside my plain trouser but then realised that there would be no privacy to remove the long-john inner thermal wear on getting to work since the changing room is unisex and shared by all and there is very little time for clothes to be removed on getting to work and putting it back on before walking home. This is another example of managers who are well paid and drive good heated cars taking decisions that hurt non-car owners and low-income earners (Carers).

Trainers footwear should be allowed

Management of care homes often as a matter of policy and dress code choose to have their Carers wearing an 'official look' in terms of attire including footwear and this decision is at the expense of the physical nature of the Carers' job. Carers are not allowed to wear trainers or canvas shoes. Considering that Carers walk several miles in total on every shift, and most of the walking involves hours of walking, running, squatting, climbing stairs up and down, walking on wet surfaces, pushing/pulling a wheelchair or hard electronically improvised fire doors, etc. These are heavily strenuous tasks that require a far greater deal of flexibility even up to the scale required by athletes. Most of the power comes from the legs and foot. Furthermore, while a Carer is assisting a resident with personal care or supporting residents to walk, there exists a serious risk and hazard of the Carer stepping on toes of the resident being assisted who will be either not wearing any shoes or wearing soft home slippers. Due to this, the sole of Carers' footwear need not be hard to prevent causing serious damage should a Carer step on a resident's foot. The soles of office shoes are far harder than canvas and trainers. Considering the above reasons, I personally think that the trainers are best suited for the job and should be allowed although colour restrictions can be applied for uniformity purposes.

Enforce rules against see-through leggings

See through leggings still being worn by female Carers especially night female Carers even though most care homes have rules against them.

It is very hard to believe that in this modern age, someone would wear see-through leggings with their knickers very clearly visible in a work environment.

In some care homes, no one seems to notice, and everyone assumes it to be normal. There are rules against them, but these rules seem very relaxed and never enforced especially in the night when worn by night female Carers.

Good quality Gloves only

Carers handle a lot more body fluid than surgeons, this warrants them receiving proper examination gloves and other personal protective equipment of highest quality. Surgical Gloves or nothing. Economically, buying the cheapest gloves for Carers leads to Carers doubling or tripling their gloves because they tore easily when soaps, water, and creams are applied and when soaked in warm water.

The CQC must ensure that all care homes provide exactly the same type and quality of glove that surgeons and doctors use to Carers as a compulsory basis because, like these medical professionals, Carers on a daily basis do handle more body fluid and are exposed to serious contaminants and infectious viruses and bacteria. It should be taken seriously to see a Carer's gloves tear while in use. CQC knows this is true but cannot be bothered to enforce it. They made SAFE (check if the care home is SAFE for residents but not Carers) part of their unannounced checks but they do not check the safety of Carers and their own health in this regard. They ask residents and relatives questions like do you feel safe living in this home but they never ask Carers questions like have your gloves ever torn or ripped while you're giving personal care or any activity that puts you in contact with an individual's body fluid?

Buy Nitrile gloves not vinyl Gloves

Vinyl gloves rip easily, therefore, they must be banned for use in all situations where body fluid is likely to be involved. CQC should ensure that no vinyl is being provided to Carers. Nitrile gloves can stretch therefore a Carer can manage to use a smaller size and securely or safely.

The amount of time to wear a double poor-quality pair of Vinyl gloves is double the time that would be spent on a single good quality pair of Nitrile gloves. I was assisting a local GP to treat a resident. He came in with his Nitrile gloves while I had on a pair of vinyl gloves provided by our care home. My gloves ripped in the middle and his gloves were OK. We were doing the exact same task and I had bodily fluid on my hands, but he did not. Why was I exposed to the risk? Because my life and health were not as important as doctors?

Gloves Sizes

Buy more large and medium gloves and less small gloves. Small gloves are used twice less than large and medium-sized gloves.

Face Masks

The face mask is a personal protective equipment PPE. It is used mainly in the medical profession. In some care homes and for certain tasks it is provided but that is less than 5% of care homes that I have been to. The world expects nursing mothers to be comfortable with their baby's faeces while giving the baby a very good thorough cleaning. It is very unfair but for real that same is expected of Carers while cleaning an elderly resident or changing stoma bags. The face masks should be provided just as gloves and other PPE are provided.

I wrote this bit long before the coronavirus epidemic, so it has nothing to do with the epidemic.

Face Splash

I have never seen this PPE ever before in all the home's I have worked in. It is a very important PPE and I do not know why they do not provide it ever. I wrote this part long before Coronavirus epidemic came.

Carers just cannot win

Routine night welfare checks and sleep disruption

Welfare checks predominantly at night times could appear from a resident's perspective to be an intrusion of privacy or nuisance as it does wake up light sleepers. Due to these reasons, some residents do not understand why it is necessary and view it as invasive. Sometimes residents react in a nasty way toward Carers during these sorts of checks and such nasty outburst does have impacts. Carers lie that they have checked all resident whereas they left out the ones who are known to seriously dislike being checked on such intervals and who have not signed undertaking that Carers should not check them maybe because their families want them to be checked or they didn't know that they can actually sign such undertaking and stop or reduce the number of times they are checked. Such nasty outburst toward Carers go unreported and the management would not be aware of the situation for a very long time and should the resident involved have a serious fall in her bedroom and the Carers would not be aware of such fall for a very long time because they have not been doing the check for fear of receiving nasty outbursts. It becomes a dilemma.

It is also worth noting that Carers do appear like perverts from perspectives of some residents because Carers when doing night routine checks, they try to quietly open each resident's door to avoid waking the resident and peep to check how the resident is doing and ensure all assisting technology and plugged in ready to use. In some cases, the resident may wake up and see a person peeping through their door, in some cases, they get frightened in which case some reassurances must be given instantly. However, the first impression is often difficult to erase especially when a new or temporary employee (Carer) is involved and sometimes due to dementia and its related memory loss, all employees

(Carers) whether old or new are new and unrecognisable by some residents.

*"**All staff at night MUST NOT take the paperwork out of the rooms!!!** All folders follow the resident at all times. If double one can tidy room and one do book. No excuses. Anyone caught bringing paper work out will be disciplined. Legal documents have been scribbled on and now are missing daily notes. Fill them out as you go along pls. Thanks*
Thanks"

The sender of this text message did not realise that to fill the forms in each room as the checks were being done means that the Carer will switch on the bedroom light and will write on a desk and flick book pages. This will also be done hourly in some cases where hourly checks are required. This, therefore, makes it impossible to not wake residents up during the checks and by waking a resident up, the Carer is disturbing the resident's sleep, therefore, creating clashes between residents enjoying sleep and Carers doing their job.

Non-smoking care home policies

It is very important that care homes create a smoking area for residents, staff and visitors to smoke their cigarettes. The idea of banning smoking within the premises is very wrong. Let me tell you a short story. Back in the old country (Nigeria), there lived a couple adjacent to a flat where I lived with my friends. They physically fought regularly and after each fight they would reflect in a quite loud manner blaming each other. On this quiet night, they had a fight, reconciled and were loudly reflecting when the wife blamed her husband's 'temperament/thin skin' on his marijuana smoking habit. She said her husband tends to fight after he must have smoked marijuana and the husband responded defending his habit and said that if not because he smoked, he would have killed her out of anger. He said that the marijuana smoking calms him down despite his wife's nagging and disrespectful behaviours. Therefore, please ban all class A, B or C drugs but do not ban cigarette smoking in care homes. Managers may encourage smokers to voluntarily smoke less or kick the habit altogether.

Staff' notices and Threats
There is very significant use of wrong words in written notices. For instance, a training announcement reads, "no attendance no work". Another occasion, "night staff must collect urine samples from the following residents", and yet another one reads, "all completed kitchen cleaning duties must be documented in the kitchen duties folder, it is not rocket science", and yet another vivid one reads, "night staff should pick up extra shifts to cover their weekly shift as it costs lot using agency staffing and not rely on the day staff to cover such shifts for them else they would be put on rota for day shift" . **"Good Evening all staff please could make sure that you are complete your notes on the pass system. if you notes are not done I will remove you from rota. If your pass system is not working please inform as soon as possible"**. First, without the Carers, there will be no care. 90% of all Management's announcements & reminders to staff on the notice board (such as training, staff meeting, keeping confidential information safe etc) have a threat and insulting comments (such as failure to comply will lead to disciplinary action or plain insulting words) attached below it which adds up to the overall treatment of staff without any integrity or respect. I can see an announcement telling staff that a new cigarette bin

was provided, and it should be used, failure to use the litter will result in the implementation of a non-smoking policy. The warning part could have been worded as, 'wouldn't you rather have a cleaner smoking area?'

The manager should ensure that only staff trained or with basic knowledge of Human Resource Management or staff who are naturally very polite can write notices on behalf of the care home administration and management.

Jack of all trades

Are they Carers or gofers?

Carers are expected to do all jobs not limited to providing personal care & support services to residents, house cleaning, cooking, making beds, shopping, organising & hosting parties/events & serving dignitaries/invitees, laundry, haircut and hairstyling, manicures & pedicures, home decorations, receptionist, administrators, drivers, activities coordinators, physiotherapist, training providers etc. Carers usually do not like but do not mind doing these tasks. The issues are that they keep multiplying and Carers are expected to do them like experts. They are expected to cook as good as cooks for instance. They are forced to undertake pieces of training originally designed for cooks and to renew or refresh their knowledge in some cases on an annual basis. But the biggest problem of all is that the Carers who by doing cooks' jobs are seen by the main cooks as being beneath them or inferior and it frustrates the cooks should a Carer get something wrong. If the Carer did not do something right, then the cook would insult the Carer and tell the Carer off or say some very degrading words to the Carer. To clarify on this, cooks work regularly in the kitchen, the cook knows exactly where the kitchen dustpan is kept or how to arrange the items in the fridge but should a Carer put the kitchen dustpan in the wrong location within the kitchen or put an item in the wrong place in the fridge, the cook would insult the Carer. If a Carer who has been told to do laundry fails to sort out the clothes properly or put cardigan in the dryer risking it shrinking, the same sort of insult would be addressed towards the Carer by the main domestic staff who sees Carers as inferior or beneath him/her when domestic duties are involved. Sometimes the domestic staff or cooks would put up a very insulting notice to communicate with Carers using phrases such as, "it's not rocket science", "Carers must", "failure to adhere means disciplinary action" as if they were the manager who can discipline any subordinate (Carers). The manager sees these notices and usually does nothing; an act which further reassures the cooks and domestic staff to continue to domineer over Carers. But it does not stop there, the next set of issues are the designation of duties to Carers as if they have not got enough duties already. In this care home, the cook was very frustrated when the dishwasher packed up, the manager simply promised to send a Carer to the kitchen after each dinner to wash up the dishes despite that 'after-dinner' is one of the busiest times as lots of toileting and transfer of residents from dining to lounges/rooms/conservatories, but problems arose when the Carer saw the cook reading magazine while she (Carer) was doing the dishes. A relative complained about the perpetually overflowing waste bin in her mother's room, what did the manager do, designate it to Carers in a very rude text message sent to all Carers telling them to ensure they empty all bins in the rooms because it is not the responsibility of the cleaners. At another time in another care home, the dryer was faulty so the night Carers didn't empty the washing machine only for the morning domestic worker to confront one of the night Carers in the morning at the end of the shift when the Carer was about going home questioning why 'common sense' didn't indicate to her to hang out the washing in radiators in corridors across the care home and they began having a serious go at each other with raised voices. This shows how often other employees look down on 'jack of all trade' Carers. The domestic staff had little understanding of infection control which prevents Carers from hanging out wet undried washings in corridors. In one care home where I worked, the cleaner starts her shift at 9:00am and finishes at 14:00 and then the Carers will be asked to do the deep cleaning tasks such as cleaning the Insect/fly trap, cooking equipment, refrigerator etc as well as other domestic tasks such as laundry and cooking. This indicates that it is a cost saving measure to get their money's worth from Carers' labour. The worse issue with this deliberate design to keep the Carers on their feet minute by minute is that they don't have the time to read and pay attention to the details of each resident's care plan and then they rely on 'hearsay' or unverified spoken pieces of information which turns out to be wrong/unreliable sometimes and most adversely, not being familiar with the locations of certain pieces of information needed by 999 operator/paramedic in times of extremely serious emergency situations. Then they get told off for taking too long to locate pieces of information in a big care plan folder or for giving wrong or partly inaccurate information to paramedics or 999 operators.

There is a danger related to this jack of all trade arrangement. On very early Christmas morning of 2019, a bank Carer was doing the laundry and loaded a duvet into the dryer, and it caused a fire. Luckily, the smoke was detected by another Carer before the fire had spread out of the dryer. She phoned fire service and began evacuation. No one was hurt and the fire was stopped by the firemen when they arrived. If Carers must do any laundry, then it should be just bedsheets and pillowcases. They are not trained to wash/dry duvet and other intricate clothes. Worse of all, an agency or a bank Carer who works only on a temporary basis may not know that duvets should be dried at different settings of the dryer, but do you blame them?

Carers being asked to fix electrical faults

I arrived at work and was having a handover. Our handover was interrupted by the day's team leader who was on call with the overall team leader discussing what to do regarding malfunctioned electrical in some bedrooms. It appears that the sister-care home's maintenance man could not be reached to attend so they were considering asking the Carers to do it and being a male Carer, I was asked to look for a screwdriver, open a wooden panel and then check out why electricity has gone out in some rooms. I refused to do it because I was angry with the management. You see, a few months ago, not because of shortage of residents or changes in rate of return, they had cut our own care home maintenance man's hours from full time down to 20 hours a week. With expectation that the maintenance man in their other care home within the company's retinue of profiteering business will also cover any overhead need at ours. Our maintenance man resigned in protest and then either they could not find any replacement due to the job offer being only a few hours or they did not bother trying to find any replacement. So now the electricity related emergency task was pushed over to Carers who were not electricians to investigate and fix. I'm not arguing that some people don't investigate and fix the same issues in their own houses where they live with their families but this is workplace and getting rid of the maintenance man in a cost saving move makes it this sort of case the director's problem and maybe he should have been phoned to come and fix it.

Home Care

Home Care Carers plight

Home Care Carers feel extremely vulnerable and they do have good reasons to be. From the children and other relatives of their clients who keep pestering them to go out with them by offering them lift, gifts etc. New Carers are most vulnerable but experienced Carers also deal with similar issues. A new Carer was tricked by a client to give him her number in case she is running late but then she ended up receiving inappropriate Sexual messages from this client. Another new Carer said on a call to support her client, the client's son kept pestering her, initially she was just being polite, and he asked her out she told him she has a boyfriend. Then on another day, he told her that he has psychic powers and her boyfriend, and she does appear incompatible from the picture he was seeing with his psychic power.

During a call, an Asian man client was doing a video call telling people on the other side of that call that he has a servant and actually turned the phone to show them the supposed servant who happened to be a Carer doing her cleaning.

In many cases, they are being bossed about by the children and spouse of their clients who aggressively want to get maximum utility like getting their money's worth but the feeling of being bossed about by someone who isn't your boss or client damages morale and causes sadness. The problem arises from managers signing care + House cleaning services agreements whereby the person being cared for shares the house with their children and retinue of relatives. A Carer who has never had any professional cleaning service training or provided professional cleaning tools will be expected to deeply clean kitchen appliances like the oven and the house and do it all in a very tightly budgeted time. A Carer will only expect his basic home knowhow from his own home is enough but, in many cases, it appears that the expectations of the retinue of relatives can only be properly met by a professional house cleaner. And one wonders why a Carer is to clean after all the people living in the house and why cannot they clean the house that they share with their relative who needs care. Why do social services pay for their house to be cleaned just because one occupant requires care?

The biggest concern is the dropping number of home care staff as well as the number of people who need home care whom the social services cannot find a home care agency because they have used almost all agencies in the area and the individual & retinue of relatives fell out with each and every one of them.

These Carers will not encourage their friends and relatives to get their sort of job.

Is striking justified in this circumstance?

Read this true scenario which happened in Leicester. A woman and her son live in a house together. The son gets a waking night Carer every night. When the Carers complained about the lack of heating in the house during the night. The issue was passed on to social workers, but nothing changed. The Carers began to contribute £10 each to the woman and the issue seemed somewhat resolved until the woman stopped putting on the heating again complaining that the £10 each of them contributes is not enough. Some Carers got angry and refused to turn up for work at that house and only then did the social workers proactively got involved to find a lasting solution to the problem. Is striking justified, I asked?

Wage commensurate with the risk

Care is just like any other healthcare very risky job. The risks include your own self-coming into contact with body fluid, the risk of making mistakes of which punishment may include prison term and risk of physical abuse by mentally challenged residents. The fact that they work with very frail and sick individuals meant that little mistake could lead to a manslaughter charge. The problem is that their wage is not commensurate with the level of this risk that they take.

Other ways to help Carers

Social care sector needs newcomers

It is very important to stop putting people off doing the job. Find a way to address their worst fears. For instance, addressing new Carers fear that it is mandatory that he or she must take part whether comfortable or not in cleaning or washing the lifeless body of a resident who passed away. That a new Carer should be allowed to wear nose and mouth cover during personal cares till they comfortably decide to stop.

One of the other sacrifices includes the fact that female Carers must never wear long nails all year round whether naturally long or artificial (fixed). Although this is an important infection prevention requirement, it adds up to the list of sacrifices amongst which continues to increase reasonable reasons why the job's attractiveness is declining. I am not advocating female Carers to wear long nails; I want their sacrifices recognised and for them to be compensated for the sacrifice by management proactively implementing best practices of Human resource management and improve the wage and welfare benefits.

Help with vouchers

Hand out free external counselling vouchers, debt management vouchers as well as quitting smoking helps & guides to your Carers.

Caregivers fatigue or personal stress/problems can only be recognised if the Carers are genuinely cared for. Take for instance, a Muslim lady working a long day during Ramadan or a lady going through menopause or even an immigrant who is seriously worried about his or her future with regards to the increasing callous anti-immigration governments. Even as I discussed earlier, a lady who works nights but due to looking after kids in the day rarely gets any sleep or pregnant lady who lost her unborn child in the summer care home heatwave.

The biggest naivety is the management expecting to be informed by the Carer going through tough times before they recognise their plight. Unfortunately, most people hide their biggest worries and try to wear a smile but dying on the inside.

I felt like adding this bit to this memoir after one colleague always comes to work hungry, always using a work shower, drinking lots of sugary fizzy drinks, smoking and eating lots of junk. I first realised that she has been doing about 250 hours each month, then I realised that she did tell me herself that she hasn't had hot water in her house for months, she also told me that she got paid over £2000 and she only had £200 left after two days and she said she was in lots of debt when I asked where her income went. She ordered takeaway the same evening and said that she has not had any meal since the previous day. She could not afford the dental treatment for her teeth and sometimes she was in lots of pain. When someone provides care services, they must be cared for. This is in the best interest of sustainable quality compassionate care.

I wrote the above piece about my colleague with severe private issues in the later part of 2019. As at now, June 2020, my colleague J.R whose life prompted me to write the above has now been off due to depression since March and counting. The company is considering telling her that they have tried waiting for her to recover and return to work but somehow, they just have not sent that letter. Our team is still hopeful that she will recover and come back to work.

Most Carers would not discuss their needs with the management or anyone that is connected to the company (employer) so for effective advice and support, a neutral and confidential third party should be regularly made available at no cost to the recipient (Carer). The October 2019 'every mind matters' campaign and advert by Public Health England, in partnership with the NHS and fronted by the Dukes and Duchesses of Cambridge and Sussex was absolutely correct; many people including Carers do face challenges to our mental health for different sorts of reasons. They feel stressed, hurting, low mood, anxious and really worried about something. Apart from things that they can do for themselves by themselves, I find it necessary to highlight things that the management can do to help.

Let's look at another issue, talking about immigration, the UK government implemented very callous anti-immigration policies for such a long time from 2012 under Home Secretary Teresa May, intensified it in 2014 under Amber Rudd and it lasted until the Windrush scandal put a sudden halt/review of the callousness. They did hurt lots of people and not just the Windrush generation. The Windrush generation scandal revealed to everyone what they had concealed for a long time; how callous they were. There's a channel called "pick" which broadcast a program titled, 'UK Border Force' and shows anti-immigration raids on public TV and sometimes it shows raids in some care homes as well as many other anti-immigration callousness and all to the amusement of some residents and some British born Carers who find it amusing while this channel is ignorantly reopening these deeply buried scars. Anyone Black Asian and Minority Ethnic [BAME] who has been through such a nightmare of immigration stress, trauma and anxiety would tell you that it leaves a deep scar. A colleague once said to me, "these people hate us" and on listening to her, I could see the scar in her mind, and it touched me.

Childcare

Nursing mums get shattered before they even arrive for a shift. The UK government has offered limited weekly childcare hours, but it appears to barely scrape the surface. I realised that a certain pregnant lady colleague of mine does not get any sleep when she returns from a night shift and returns to work later in the evening for another night. Then she takes lots of tobacco and red bull to keep going.

The long school holidays in the UK is most difficult for Carers and care homes as kids are spending their holidays, their parents need to give them 24 hours and this affects the parent's work-life balance

Children Holiday

Carers like to spend the holiday with their children when their school terms are over. This brings increased demand for Carers holidays to correspond with the children holiday and it becomes a dilemma when there are few Carers with children and all asking for a holiday at the same time. Childcare costs spiral out of control for the Carers since the kids will need some childcare whenever they are at home. Care home management should act as a cooperative society and negotiate cheap childcare or subsidise it for the Carers because if the cost of childcare surpasses wage, then work becomes less important. It is in managers best interest.

Avoid Scorched earth policies

The term scorched earth policy according to Cambridge dictionary is the military policy of destroying anything that the enemy might value while advancing or retreating troops from locations in enemy or own territory. You may wonder if this sort of policy exists in care homes today and to your greatest surprise, it does exist. So, you see why such policies are not for some compassion-based environment like care homes. For instance, when listing tasks that you expect to be completed by the end of a shift, try not to make it looks like on behalf of the directors, that like a scorched earth policy, you are trying to squeeze out as much work as possible out of Carers in order to get your money worth in terms of economic maximum utility of labour force. Do not ever give such an impression as you do not want to see any Carer idle or sitting down. Avoid taking such a position as if all chores are done, the Carers can help mown the lawn. Instead, if you see a Carer sweating, encourage that Carer to go outside with a cold drink and return after 15 minutes (paid) cooling down time. This is not for managers and seniors alone, it should be explained to certain residents who assume Carers are servants or maids and dislike to see an idle Carer because such residents genuinely do exist and as soon as they see a Carer idle, they would begin to think of an errand to send the Carer on. Sometimes this is heightened by a resident's failure to notice that the team of Carers are understaffed and were still expecting all their demands and requests met in entirety. This raises the stress levels significantly driving Carers faces into frowning mode.

Managers and senior Carers, please do not use words like 'Must', or in any way threaten the Carers with disciplinary action should they fail to complete tasks designated or decline to pick up extra shifts to cover other sick colleagues. Although laziness is condemned, it is the manager's duty to evaluate the stress levels. Another good instance of scorched earth policy is the 'Bin excess food' policy is scorched earth policy.

I have been on a day shift at this local council owned home in 2014, Carers fed residents and then it appears that the kitchen cooks prepare more food than needed. To my surprise, the cooks were instructed that all excess food must be discarded, and no staff is to be allowed to have any, even if they are to have it only while on break in the staff room. In another care home, I received the following message from the administrator's office, "It has come to our attention that people are not paying for their meals. This will now be closely monitored, and meals will be thrown away if not paid up front

Thanks

Admin"

I was very sad upon reading this message. The management was threatening to discard leftover food if Carers do not pay. The cost of each leftover plate is £0.50 pence and if Carers do not pay for it then it will be discarded, and it made me question if it is worth it really? In the same care home, there is a banner on the wall that reads, "residents don't live at our workplace, we work at their home". This quote is only true and practical if the organisation and its residents live up to it by treating the Carers nicely. Would you discard food at your own home when there is a hungry individual with you at the time?

The funny thing is that there is a certain relative who visited daily and usually had meals at no cost with her mother who was our resident. Some Carers always murmured why they had to pay for dinner but she (visiting relatives) was not.

The damage to compassionate care which this wicked message would cost the management is far more than fifty pence. What can fifty pence buy the care home? This sort of policy of rather throwing your excess extra food to spare away into the bin rather than give it to your exhausting Carers who may not have brought a pack up with them to work is hypocritical of your management begging Carers to pick up extra shifts from their extra time to spare.

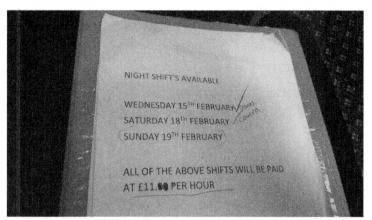

NIGHT SHIFT'S AVAILABLE

WEDNESDAY 15TH FEBRUARY
SATURDAY 18TH FEBRUARY
SUNDAY 19TH FEBRUARY

ALL OF THE ABOVE SHIFTS WILL BE PAID
AT £11.00 PER HOUR

Have you ever wondered why even when you offer £2.00 extra for any extra shifts, none of your Carers would want to cover it still? I recalled a Carer who after a 12 hours day shift, one of the night Carers didn't turn and the recruitment agencies that were contacted had no Carer to send out so a day Carer volunteered to do a night shift after she had just completed a 12 hour shift and the following week, she also received that wicked text message about 0.50 pence.

Asking a Carer who has not got food in front of him to encourage a resident to eat is silly. There is no resonance effect. My physics teacher tried several times to explain resonance and many students were left behind until he explained that resonance is similar to the feeling you get when you are walking somewhere with your friends and suddenly some of them wants to go to the men's or ladies room and you end up going with them and having a pee even though you didn't feel like having one earlier. What better way would Carers encourage residents who are not good eaters hence losing lots of weight than to eat side by side with the resident at mealtimes.

Strictly avoiding any other way of Killing compassion should be taken seriously. Show compassion to your staff and they may reciprocate.

Clarify what staff are/are not allowed to eat/drink

To avoid this issue that occurs every care home that I have been to, it would be helpful if the management would clarify what staff are allowed to eat/drink and what they are not allowed to eat/drink and permanently post it on the kitchen or staff room notice boards. It is very embarrassing for any Carer to be told that they have had food that they are not allowed to have. It kills compassionate care so the earlier and permanently this information is put up, the better for everyone.

Free Wi-Fi

Care Homes should give their Carers free Wi-Fi when they are on break. Considering that Carers are not allowed to leave the premises even during their break and also considering that they need to contact their families who may be based in a different continent or country via video/audio calls or other Internet-based communication media and lastly considering that most Internet broadband in the UK is unlimited data usage so it will not add any extra costs to the company. This is one of the little ways to show Carers that you (management) does care. When you see a manager strictly hiding the broadband password from Carers it somehow sends a message of 'hate' or contempt to the Carers. In this Carer home I worked was so remote that there's no mobile wireless network available but the fibre optic broadband landline is connected and there is Wi-Fi in the building but I made up my mind to never work there again because there is no way to communicate with my loved ones because they will not give Carers the broadband access.

Pay wages before big sales

Here are more ideas on how to make your Carers happier and feel appreciated,

Instead of a manager sending this sort of message out, "None of you are down for the Christmas night out....... Can I motivate any of you?!". There are a lot of ways to motivate the Carers. The last payday before Christmas is usually on the last working day of November whereas there are 'Black Friday' sales which take place before this payday. Based on several conversations, many Carers will be very grateful if they can be paid a day before Black Friday or Boxing day sales event. Carers are on a low-income level of earnings so therefore they will need to have the cash to take advantage of the massive Black Friday sales to buy the much-needed Christmas presents for their loved ones and the boxing day sales too. This will be very much appreciated by the Carers and is quite another brilliant way to appreciate them. Maybe if they feel appreciated, then they may put their name down and attend the company's Christmas night out or any other get together to celebrate a successful year.

Xmas Party Budget could be put to better use
Since the biggest concern for most of the staff during the Xmas and New year period is logistics. Most people worry about how they will get to work and how they will get home. There will be no bus service for those who rely on the bus service. The taxi companies will charge a fare and a half of a fare on Xmas eve, boxing day and on new year eve and then double fare on Xmas day and new year day. And, since it is very likely that due to several reasons not limited to ill-treatment of staff by the management, most of the staff would likely boycott the end of year staff party. In my humble opinion, it would be good to calculate the cost of each seat of the table (I assume that you will take them out to eat before going elsewhere to a party) and offer the staff cash to help with taxi fares. Alternatively, give them a choice or vote for what they want; spend half of the end of year

party fund on a taxi for those who don't want a party but need taxi fare costs covered and the other half for those who drive to go on and party.

12 or more hours shift patterns and staff rooms

It is very cruel of directors and managers to have Carers work 12 hours shift or more and not have any serene (frigate/mess/staffroom) place to retreat to on interval during the 1-hour unpaid break that they usually get. Since they will not be allowed to leave the property during their unpaid break, they should be encouraged to get as much relaxation as possible within this break hour. It should be essential that there should not be any call bell notifier in this staffroom even for emergency purposes. The new level low currently existing in care homes or are being introduced now requires Carers to work 12 hours day shifts and 12 hours night shifts and new employees are questioned or scrutinised if they can and are willing to do this sort of shift pattern before they are offered care assistant jobs because they will be told during interview that it is the only shift pattern available. I am not against this shift pattern but there must be choices of other lesser hours available and it should not be mandatory or be the only shift pattern available. The funny bit is, if given the job, then the Carer will be given a document by the employer to sign that he or she accepts to work beyond the health and safety executive recommended daily working hours as if the Carer genuinely chose to. The health and safety executive requires employers to ensure that workers working beyond the recommended daily hours genuinely choose to do so and can manage and reduce stress level during each long shift. If they are forced to work 12 hours or more in a stretch, at least, a well-planned staffroom is not just important, it should be mandatory for all care homes to provide one. Carers need a staff room with equipment to wash hands, warm up their pack up food and refrigerator to cool their refreshments. A toilet, dining table and comfortable sofa. There should not be any call bell in the staff room and if they are required to abandon the break and attend to emergency situations, then their break should be paid breaks and they should be considered to be "on-call". There should not be any camera CCTV in staff rooms since this is their private time. Access to their phone and gadgets should be allowed so that they can contact families and friends.

In this care home where a staffroom, kitchenette and toilet were provided for staff in the staffroom area, I could not help but notice that the area never gets cleaned by the domestic staff. I once asked a domestic staff why they never cleaned the staff toilet and to my surprise she said that it is not part of their job to clean the staff room and the toilet. Worst thing was that when the care home appeared to be running out of space, they started storing things in the staff toilet. Things such as a standing fan which will only be needed in summer, mop buckets & utensils, 3 big leftover paint buckets with paint contents and an out of use shower chair. These render the staff toilet unused due to lack of space.

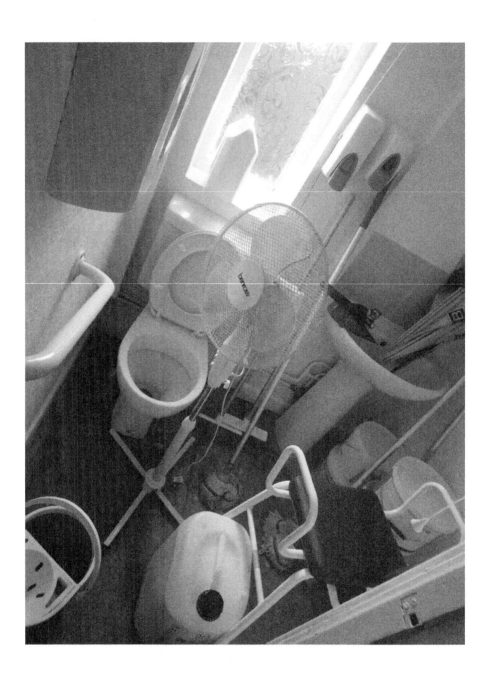

Most painful of them all

To make matters worse, when the nurses refrigerator (located in the medication storage room & used to store medicines at required temperature) packed up, our manager had an urgent need to collect a resident's faeces and urine samples and preserve them at fridge temperature until they get delivered to the GP/laboratory for test. The manager stored these in the staff room's refrigerator, and we found out when we went on break to have our meals.

These wicked acts are part of subconscious tendencies to look down on Carers, overlook them, neglect them and consider them as irrelevant. These bad attitudes often take its toll on the level of compassionate care that exists in the care home.

Observed Carers' reaction to 'no staffroom'

Having no staff room provided for the Carers, there is a little part of the dining room that is a bit elevated like a stage and in the middle was the Victorian fireplace with two adjacent lounge chairs. On the floor down the rest of the dining room are the normal dining chairs and tables. I observed on my first day how Carers would during their breaks, trying to improvise then turned the two adjacent lounge chairs to face the wall so that when they sit down to enjoy their break, they will be completely have turned their backs on the rest of the building and that exactly what one of the Carers said when I teased her about how rude she seems to turn her back on the dining room where I was sitting having my break with two residents who both had dementia and kept on asking me for assistance and to explain over and over why they were living in the care home. I could have served them better if I got that moment of serenity and rejuvenation which break times should be designed to offer to Carers and then continuing where I left off to give reassurances. Another issue is that, since the dining room is usually the only vacant room for staff to stay and have their mid-morning breaks since no staffroom is provided but then the cleaners need to mop the floor with bleach or other toxic chemicals after breakfast to clean up spills and foods and sterilise the floor of the dining room. With Carers having their breaks and inhaling beech because they have no alternative. This is terribly wrong.

Carers' break times routinely interrupted

A colleague angrily narrates her ordeal. She said because there is no staffroom, she was having her break in the dining room behind the entrance door with her phone and drink. A relative walked up to her and asked for her help to make drinks for her mum and her other sister who were also visiting. My colleague said that it would be rude to tell her to ask someone else for help because she was on break, so she interrupted her break and made them all cups of tea. The relative a few minutes later went down to the office and complained that she was unhappy having to come down to request for her mum to have drinks while she could see a Carer "idly sitting down on her phone having a drink". My colleague was summoned to the office immediately to explain why she was on her phone having a drink and this summoning interrupted her break for the second time. And hearing that despite making the relatives drink, they still were not satisfied, made her feel very sad. My colleague went on to describe how relatives and residents who have dementia will always interrupt her breaks. Residents with dementia will walk up to her asking over and over what time or day it is. All these happen because there is not a staffroom and neither the CQC nor safeguarding team of the local council cares.

Dry hands

The most important part of the hygiene system in care homes is washing of hands on a regular basis. It is therefore surprising to notice that few impediments to hand washing are often ignored. A good example is the non-provision of lotions for Carers to use and prevent dry hands which will likely occur from too frequent hand washing with chemicals. Care Homes and the regulatory bodies still do not see the duty of care to protect Carers and at the same time promote regular hand wash to boost hygiene.

Unhealthy work environment and recycling

Kitchen and Medical waste recycling

The CQC should as part of their unannounced inspection check out care homes recycling and waste disposal policy and systems. In all care homes that I have worked, 95% of them do not separate recyclable plastic from other waste. They pay good attention to ensuring yellow bags and outdoor bins are provided for faecal and other body fluid. They also strictly provide required disposal for drugs and needles/syringes and to my astonishment, they do not provide bins for recyclables. This is because they will have to pay for its collection. This is no omission, rather it is a premeditated decision. They must be forced to stop it. As at this moment June 2018, Carers put recycle bins in their homes so that their families would put recyclables in correct bins but then when they get to work, they are forced to put recyclables in the wrong bins. This is wrong and a crime against humanity and sustainable living.

Caring is essential and it is not just caring for residents. The company must care for the environment and the staff as well as for their own selves. Disregard for the environment by not caring to provide recycling bins for whatever reason is totally sending the wrong signal that they do not care.

One of my biggest upsets was a local Food Standards Agency rating of a care home; 5 out of 5 even though they did not have any recycling practices such as segregation of waste or isolation of recyclable wastes. They mix plastics and other food waste together in the kitchen and did not care to provide a different bin for recycling and yet the hygiene agency rated them 5.

There is currently zero move to sort medical waste in care homes beyond syringes and expired tablets. Gloves and incontinent pads are dropped into the same yellow bin bags. It would not be difficult to create a very distinctly designed care home bins that will help keep the wastes sorted. It is true that there are yellow bags and black bags provided but there is usually no system for recycling medical related plastic waste.

Plastic bin liners

Save the planet, use as few plastics as possible. Carers who care for the planet do not like the idea of white plastics in all lounge bins and at the end of the day, a very large amount of plastic is used in care homes.

Care homes use an awful number of plastic bags every day and there are several ways to cut this. But in some cases, it is very essential for infection control reasons, then a good recycling policy should be followed so that care homes use only recycled plastics.

Prevent unhealthy working environment?

Do Carers who do not smoke have the right to be protected by law or care agencies mandated to offer Carers the choice to refuse to work in residents' rooms or homes if the residents smoke in their rooms or bungalow or conservatory especially in airtight sort without proper ventilation? Or if the environment is generally unhealthy?

This problem relates more to home Carers who look after residents in their own homes. This is because most care homes are either smoke free or have smoking lounges. But should Carers be mandated to spend time in smoking lounges in care homes even if they do not wish to?

I was asked to attend to a gentleman in his bungalow. On getting there, the entire house was full of cigarette smoke and since it was a supported living arrangement, he was at low risk of fire but the house was very full of cigarette stench and very difficult to breathe for me throughout my stay in his house and when I got out the clothes I wore bore the stench of cigarette mixed up with steam which smells so bad that I felt embarrassed and unhappy. I think Carers should have the right to be forewarned, to refuse to attend to a certain poorly designed smoking environment especially where adequate ventilation is lacking. The problem is that if a Carer speaks up and declined to help a resident due to the environmental situation related to resident's airtight smoking, the manager or team leader may misunderstand it as Carer being difficult or mean or lazy or stubborn or simply put 'bad attitude to work' and this puts Carers off speaking up but then holding a grudge or being sad while in the middle of a job doesn't achieve any compassionate care and does no good to anyone. Although it is the resident's house and the resident can do whatever he or she likes in their own house they must consider non-smokers who will be coming in to assist them and spending about an hour or more in there. The Law against smoking in bus stops should apply here.

Pollution
Care homes are the most polluted places to live. Most serious is the noise. We have on average 2 lounges and a conservatory, each having its own radio or television which is always turned on from morning till night time and poor architectural reasons the lounges and conservatory are all next to each other connected with double doors which are open all day and all night. Considering that some residents struggle with their hearing, these appliances' volumes are always turned up louder than average. Besides, there is usually a radio in the kitchen, dining and administration office which adds to the noise. The problem is that care homes do not have a well thought through (planned) noise control policy and therefore, the volumes of these appliances can go up unchecked.

At night times, the call bells are far too loud for the residents and this results in situations where one resident presses the call bell for assistance and the bell's noise waking lots of other residents up.

I raised the noise pollution with my manager during one staff meeting and she dismissed it with the reason being that everyone has to get used to it because some residents have poor hearing and other residents have dementia while another resident has a medical condition and only enjoys constantly jingling music instruments loudly. I still felt that it was not fair to see a resident sitting in the lounge with both hands covering ears.

Loud banging by the care home's fire doors

Over time, it clearly sounds normal that many care homes' doors do not close gently without a loud bang and it appears that no one notices any more, not even the maintenance staff. The main reason for the bang is that they are fire doors, and have an instrument installed on them to ensure that they return to closed positions after it has been opened. The bang wakes residents up at night. Carers are very busy with work and most of the doors are quite heavily pushing towards being shut. These reasons are why Carers do not hold the doors to force it to shut gently without any bang. It adds up to the noise pollution of care homes. I am not a trained maintenance staff, but I believe that there must be some way of reducing the impact while ensuring that fire doors automatically close as required. It also puts a strain on the Carers who must hold these heavy doors for residents to pass through. The funny bit is that some residents have no idea how heavy fire doors could be and when a Carer is struggling to hold the door and at the same time trying not to stand in the way of the resident whose job is to walk through the door, some residents would at that point pause to rest before continuing the walk and when the Carer say please walk through quickly because this door is heavy, the resident's old age related deafness makes this communication ineffective and the Carer would repeat it many times while holding this heavy door and standing in an unbalanced position. Managers and maintenance personnel should pay attention to this.

Nuisance Social Media workgroups

If it is well regulated, it will be alright but when you have every member acknowledging a message received with an "ok" reply and your phone blowing up with endless notifications. It feels like I have brought work home to my bed when I was not even on call. But even for a manager who is on call still needs to be contacted only when it is important, there's a need to keep a phone on high alert because urgent calls may come in so no mute must be put on the phone. It must be reduced to the nearest minimum. Only relevant messages should be sent. No need for each member to acknowledge or there is no need to set up a social media group in the first place since we all meet at work weekly. If a social media group must be set up, then people should be shown how to mute or turn off notifications for the group only. Then people who do not use WhatsApp or who do not wish to join the group for whatever reason deserve to get any information that is considered relevant as well.

Insect infestation

This is a very serious matter since Insects act as a vector for spreading disease-causing microorganisms. The problem is serious in the Summer season and very difficult to control. All care homes should have an Insect net on windows and main entrance. The other side of the problem occurs in September and

October when the care homes experience some sort of Spider infestation and it appears that there are not any insect inhibitors or traps for spiders so they multiply.

Fireworks and Bonfire nights
Care homes dread this day as it increases the anxiety and induces fear in some residents. But the fact that this night or day will happen at least in the next foreseeable future. I was surprised and at the same time deep down afraid of something going wrong when our manager tried something unheard of which was to advertise on the activities board that we were to have fireworks displays in the car park as soon as sunset on November 5th and we did and it was thoroughly safe, enjoyed by many residents who wore their entire warmth clothing and they were excited. Other residents were watching from their bedroom windows and had lots of smiles on their faces. This approach could be emulated.

Palliative care and bereavement

Wake keeping should be on a voluntary basis

Care homes' policy and procedures prevent Carers from having any close attachment with any resident yet in a particular extreme case, a Carer who had no emotional attachment would be asked to keep wake/vigil and sit next to a dying resident and to hold his hand in some cases.

In this care home, a resident was on end of life and we could all see that the resident was likely to pass away that night or the following day. Since none of his relatives bothered to stay beside him, our senior Carer on shift who was in charge that night requested that we should all go and sit with him through the night. She made it mandatory. I declined to do that and rather suggested that we did more regular observations on the resident and to provide all required care to the resident. She did not like my suggestion and to my surprise, I felt so much like my suggestion came across her like I am a hater and do not care about the residents. I later felt vindicated when on another night, another colleague of mine was complaining that she was told to sit on the bedside of another resident who was dying and to hold his hand.

These stipulations are very unfair to the Carers because it should not be mandatory.

Washing deceased residents

They are Carers, not undertakers and must not be forced to wash any resident deceased while waiting for undertakers to come or while waiting for the doctors to pronounce them dead. It is fine to ask for volunteers to help do it, but it must be made explicitly clear that if the Carer is not comfortable, then the Carer does not have to.

The interim funeral home plan must be available

I have seen far too many situations where relatives argue over which funeral home/directors to contact their loved one's deceased body. This results in the deceased body remaining in the care home for unreasonable amounts of time after a doctor's confirmation of death and issuing an authorization to contact funeral directors. The Care Home should be allowed by CQC to appoint an interim and neutral funeral home from where the relatives can take the body from.

Seek out each resident's relatives while alive

In mid-2019, we lost one of our residents. The last time she had a visitor was five years ago. She died in hospital. The social services, police and the management could not find any of her kin. They all tried their very best. In the end, we, being her last people on earth, had to encourage ourselves to attend her funeral and pay our respects. Her ashes were kept in the garden of the care home.
This prompts me to add the experience to this Memoir, the need to seek residents' kin while they were alive and endeavour to keep in touch at least twice a year. This must be part of the resident's care plan and not just because it is necessary at the time of death but also it is part of healthy living for a resident to keep in touch with a relative.

A day before the funeral date, our new young manager was suspended and on the day of the funeral, she resigned. She was meant to book a taxi for staff members whom she talked into agreeing to attend the funeral held at 9:30am but her absence on that particular day meant that only two staff members attended one of whom was a night Carer who had finished a night shift and waited till 9:30am to attend. Obviously, it was this close to being that no one attended this lady's funeral. Two months after writing this part of the memoir, the deceased resident's daughter phoned asking after her mother. She was told the sad news of her death. Her mother's ashes have not been disposed of because no one knew where to dispose of it, so it was still in the office. She came and collected it together with her mother's few belongings. About two months later, I saw a bereavement card and asked my colleague who sent it, then I was told it was from the ward where she spent her last days at our Care home.

Critical issues

Should moving into a care home mean no Sex life?

One evening, my colleague narrated to us about an incident where a male resident reached for her boobs. She was not very upset about it at the time of this discussion probably because it was a few minutes before the shift was over and we were excited to be going home to rest. But it prompted us to discuss a rarely discussed issue, should a resident's sex life end the moment he or she moves into a care home? Five of us deliberated on it. First, we challenged each of us to mention a resident that we know who have had sex since that resident moved into a care home and none of us can think of one. We even thought about younger residents in their 50s. Then, we analysed what one of us said, 'it's due to their ages' and agreed that age isn't the issue since we have two residents who were in their fifties but live in our home due to Multiple Sclerosis and Parkinson diseases respectively who don't have any sex life and we also agreed that even a ninety-year-old individual may still want to have sex. We also discussed that most of our residents' partners are dead but we agreed that there is no reason why a resident who can afford an 'escort' should be denied one if the resident requests to have one phoned on his or her behalf. We further discussed if there is any escort with DBS or Police clearance and checks certificate to guarantee the safety of residents. Then we discussed the word, 'request'. We agreed that it would take a serious deal of boldness for any resident to walk up to the manager's office and say, 'phone me an escort for tonight or today'. Why is it so? We asked ourselves. We jokingly said it is probably why the gentleman reached for the lady's boobs. Returning to our discussion, we asked, why residents' relatives, management, residents themselves and all other stakeholders do not talk about this issue and we all agreed that if residents are starved of sex, then it is not fair even if they don't talk about it and we agreed that this has to change since it is not normal.

A care home cannot be a home away from home if certain things are completely ruled out by circumstances of no one doing. We concluded that the management and relatives should engage residents in such a discussion to encourage them to open and provide them with choices or options available. it is wrong that it is virtually impossible to access information on how to navigate the Care home setting, privacy, resident's continuous sex life and relationships while living in the Care home.

Quite a few residents of both sexes masturbate and by doing so they fiddle with their incontinent pad and push it out of position and thereby rendering it irrelevant and still gets soaked. It is important that this is taken into consideration so that a different type of incontinent pad is supplied, for example the pull up which automatically returns to its position even when pushed or shifted. In one shift at a care home, my colleagues were discussing and being against a certain male resident who was always watching 'Babe station' adult TV after midnight and depriving himself of sleep and they were not allowed to switch his tv off and they weren't happy. One lady said she felt like it was sexual abuse against her to be in his room providing drink while he was watching another naked woman. I said to her that she can ask me (a male) to send his tea next time but she needs to let him live his life the way he likes since everything else (lost his wife, house, independence etc.) had been taken away from him.

Stingy Lorazepam

Before we go deeper, let me share this true story. A resident was becoming too violent towards her Carers during personal care and other supports. The Enabling Research in Care Homes

(ENRICH) also known as the 'ENRICH TEAM' were informed and they came to assess her to see what needs doing. They arrived at the care home when the lady was asleep in her bed and insisted that she was not woken up to avoid her getting agitated. The staff wanted her to be seen exhibiting the same behaviour that the ENRICH team are preventing. It then appeared to the staff that the ENRICH team did not want to help for whatever reason they had, they did not see any urgency in the situation as the staff had felt, rather the ENRICH team from their action want things to remain the way they were which in other words, meant that they did not care whether staff were being physically assaulted each time they went to assist the lady with personal care.

I have always called a tablet used to calm residents down when they become very anxious and violent beyond a reasonable level. I call it 'stingy Lorazepam' because the senior Carers who do medication are strictly forbidden from giving this tablet except when it is very clearly necessary. This instruction is extremely observed to a point where this tablet is given after a preventable incident has occurred. Such an incident as a resident hitting a staff, visitors or fellow residents. Sometimes when Carers inform the senior Carer or nurse in charge of giving out medication that a particular resident who has Lorazepam prescription is very unsettled or is provoking other residents, the senior or nurse who usually sitting in the administration office hence lacking first-hand knowledge of the fast developing situation in the lounge or conservatory but would keep Lorazepam on the stingy side until the situation has developed into an incident. The resident will refuse to take the tablet at this time and the more a nurse attempts to persuade an already agitated resident to take a tablet that he or she has refused to take increases the resident's agitation and still the tablet remains highly unlikely to be taken. Lorazepam at that condition can be considered a failed option and for a very long time because the resident will now be required to be protected by one or two Carers depending on level of agitation or aggressive behaviour despite the fact that in most cases, the local council has no package for a one-to-one care for the resident so this leaves the rest of the care team seriously understaffed. This will be happening daily. In some instances, Lorazepam may be ineffective, and this went on for months until a serious incident occurred. Only then did they review his medication and mental state and then prescribed the risperidone which settled his mind and helped his anxiety because it was given mornings and evenings rather than [when needed] when he was clearly kicking off.

Should lounge seats be reserved or not?

Care Home's sitting policies should always be well highlighted in every lounge. I do admit that management's policies of no one owning any chairs does not work sometimes because we humans are territorial animals and would fight for whatever we deemed to be ours or accustomed to and in this circumstance, lounge chairs. Whatever policy that the management chooses [whether to allocate chairs or keep all chairs on a first come first served basis] should be clearly and visibly indicated in each lounge like a wall clock. This is another one of such issues brushed under the carpet like it does not exist or it is not much of a problem despite its severe consequences such as regular exchange of words by residents over lounge chairs.

Areas of further research and invention

Anti-slippery Slippers

Residents wearing slippery Slippers make standing up from the lounge chairs more difficult.

Bring the sound nearer to the chairs

To help reduce noise pollution in care homes, it may help to develop a better system that brings the sounds closer to the chairs where residents are sitting in a more targeted approach than indiscriminate sounding from TVs which pollute the environment.

A portable mobile electronic gadget that Carers can communicate with each other with, get call bell notifications, connectable to main WIFI systems and computers, camera, reminders of residents' repositioning or observations when due or other duties, face recognition of residents and able to provide on the spot information such as if they are diabetic or swallowing issues or for accurate medication, connectable to wireless earpiece in one ear, automatically turns itself off or on standby to avoid contamination, GPS connectable and recordable to trace whereabouts of each Carer within the building and throughout the shift, connectable to a video calling a resident or other staff.

Hearing aid: These are very expensive and highly unprotected items, due to Dementia, some residents fiddle with them and quickly they get lost. Carers do not like items of such cost going missing because before you (relative) even get to point fingers, the Carers already feel bad. Eyeglasses have loops on which prevents falling off. The hearing aid needs a bit more security to prevent loss or to aid detection like a remote-controlled vibration or laser flashing.

Care Home upholstery and recliner chairs require further research in terms of ease of cleaning it up when soaked on body fluid or drinks. Leathers are cold and are not very skin friendly but cotton or polyester based upholstery materials absorb stain or are very difficult to clean and maintain. Imagine a resident who has loose bowel on a cotton sofa, that is a good idea of the sort of very serious bacteria that cotton sofas could harbour.

Low lounge chairs
Lounge chairs being low hinders residents from standing up easily especially after sitting down for a couple of hours. It is also very uncomfortable to sit in a tall lounge chair, so it is necessary for the lounge chairs to be able to go up and down just like a recliner but at far cheaper cost than the recliner.

Anti-spill urine bottle
Replace the paper based single-use urine bottles with longer lasting, anti-spill metal or plastic urine bottles. The paper urine bottles are not environment friendly because they quickly go soggy and get thrown away.

Beds
Hospital beds should have space for drinking water or beakers just as seen on dashboards to prevent spillage. Residents who are bed bound should be treated like a car driver who will spend hours sitting in the driver's seat driving. The bed should have space for remote control, another space for a mug or beaker etc.

Elevated toilet seats/stand aid
The only modification that currently exists to help elderly people to use modern toilets is the elevated toilet seats which aid residents to stand up easily after using the toilet. For ladies, this

is a fantastic and effective modification. For the gentlemen, a huge failure considering that most elderly men have prostate enlargement and other prostate-related medical issues which means that they will regularly go to the toilet to urinate and urinate on the floor. This occurs because the toilet seat elevator and its pivot legs prevent the gentlemen from walking closer and standing nearly directly above the toilet to urinate. In other normal non-modified toilets, it is already difficult for gentlemen to urinate without any urine dropping on the floor or toilet bowl ring. In most observations that I carried out, the urine falls on the toilet seat elevator and then goes to the floor. In bedrooms with toilet facility, this gives their bedroom a constant pungent smell of urine. The cleaners try but in most care homes, they do not actually carry out very deep cleaning and since they clean the bedroom once per 24 hours, the pungent smell becomes unavoidable.

When a male resident sits down on an elevated toilet seat, due to the fact that this toilet seat elevator reduces the diameter of the bowl coupled with the fact that the enlarged prostate condition may exist, their penis will not face down into the toilet, it will drop on the seat and urine will still flow down onto the floor. The third issue is that the toilet seat elevator confuses many male dementia residents as it changes the look of a toilet and without prompting, they would be in the toilet but they will not be able to recognise it and still urinate on the floor or hand wash sink or toilet bin. The toilet seats harbour germs because it hides several areas where urine drops and such areas are unreachable without first dismantling the toilet seat elevator and when toilets are flushed, the water cleans the main toilet but does not clean the elevated seat.

I will recommend that ladies have their own toilet while gentlemen have theirs. This will reduce the rate of complaints and upset that ladies feel when they see urine on toilet seats. The CQC should enforce this.

I will also recommend that since the size of the toilet seat elevator and its pivot legs prevent the gentlemen from walking closer and standing nearly directly above the toilet even when staff encouraged them to do so. I recommend that gents have a toilet for defecating and a different toilet designed for urination.

Redesign the pad to withstand the washing machine

The industry has tried telling Jack-of-all trade Carers to remember to remove any incontinent pad that may be hidden in a pile of clothes before loading them into the washing. This has not worked and each week the incontinent pad will burst while in the washing machine and ruin many clothes, release lots of fluff in the drier and increase fire risk. The makers of these pads if they are reading this can try to make the pads stronger to withstand the washing machine.

Ease finding lost hearing aid

The hearing aid is an expensive medical instrument and quite small. It goes missing every day when you put the nature of the resident using it into consideration you would understand why. There are remote controls that I have seen that can reveal its own location whenever it goes missing. Similar technology should be adapted to the hearing aid to probably use Bluetooth or laser or sound to reveal its location if it is missing.

CQC & other government agencies

Standardisation of Room, corridors and elevators sizes

As a matter of safety, there should be a standard size of the room where the occupant resident requires hoisting even if the resident requires hoisting only sometimes but not all time. Lots of accident occur as a result of poorly planned care homes especially in listed buildings from Edwardian or Victorian days which have been converted into a care home without adequate thought given to the difficulty manoeuvring equipment and safety of residents. This should be part of CQC inspection. Carers are seriously struggling to manoeuvre hoists around extremely confined spaces with rug carpets, crash mats, bed motor cables and items of furniture impeding every action to manoeuvre. Corridors are too small. Lifts can barely contain a Carer and a resident in a wheelchair. Bad decisions to grant licence for such buildings to be used for care home purpose is usually taken by people who never done care in their lives. Maybe a few of them have managed a care home but it is very different from doing the job. Worst is that should an accident occur, the Carers get blamed.

CQC should adopt Ramsay's Approach

I first heard of the words, 'management contract' when the UK Conservative government was stepping in to sort out the failing Northern Rail franchise in October 2019. It involves creating an arrangement under which the government or its chosen representative enterprise oversees Northern Rail's operational control. This option of management contract was weighed against complete government renationalisation.

The CQC should go further than being a regulatory and observer commission to set up another allied agency that will focus solely on helping failing homes make and sustain all recommended improvements. If a man called Ramsey can revamp failing restaurants in America as seen on TV, then the CQC can send a highly trained staff to spend one month with critically failing homes and help the home bounce back. Teach them the way to do it from care plan creation to human resource management to customer service to etc and at the same time pay attention to the business side and protect the investor's interests. Whether CQC should force them to pay for this service is not for me to advise. This agency should on its own run a consultancy service for directors to comfortably seek their intervention when things are seemingly going bad rather than wait till the CQC has visited. The same agency should help train managers during their stay to ensure sustainable development and run of the home.

Increase CQC key questions

CQC inspects care homes to ensure that they are 1. Effective, 2. caring, 3. safe, 4. Responsive and 5. well-led. This should be increased to contain 6. care staff welfare.

This is in line with my notion that until you care for Carers and implement best practices of human resources management, compassionate care or person-centred care would remain nothing but an illusion.

For instance, I worked at a care home that scored exceptionally well in CQC inspections but has no restroom for staff and staff must share a toilet with residents. There is a CCTV camera installed in the basement where staff are expected to hang their jackets, so they are being watched even when they are changing into work clothes.

It's not as if the care homes cannot convert one of their numerous bedrooms into a staff room, rather, it's a matter of choice, a bad choice to pay less attention and care even less for the care staff and with full attention given to the rate of return on investment. CQC need to check among other things like welfare of Carers, Check the quality of PPE provided for their protection, analyse several sickness calls per month and how many were due to bad backs among other welfare specific packages.

Don't expect Carers to bite the finger that feeds them by telling you about their poor working conditions, rather do your own observations without interviewing the Carers on welfare subjects and to avoid reprisals should they tell you that they are not looked after. There should be a list of boxes to tick and care homes scored in terms of the welfare of their staff team.

On inspection day

CQC conducted an inspection while I was on a day shift, firstly, they failed to notice that our manager as soon as she heard that CQC was around, picked up the phone and called three extra staff and convinced them to come in despite they're not being on the rota and soon they joined us. The CQC agents did not record the number of staff that they saw when they arrived. Secondly, their presence meant that we were unable to take any break in the morning and we only had a break after 7 hours because we dare not take any break when the residents kept on demanding for this and that and we resiliently continued to meet these demands ensuring everything is as perfect as possible even at the expense of ourselves. The CQC did not notice that none of the Carers had had any break. Does the CQC agents care about care staff at all one must ask. Why must their entire focus be on the care that residents received? The CQC report was very impressive because the Carers overworked and overstressed themselves, but it is totally unsustainable since they will not work like that every day and the staffing numbers will drop soon as CQC officials leave.

Carers must not be questioned during CQC inspections

CQC inspections were ongoing, early in the morning of the second day before the CQC agents had arrived, our manager knew we would be interviewed later in the day by the CQC agents so she tried to convince us to watch what we say. She spoke for over 15 minutes and at the end, she said that she was not asking us to lie but then you can question what she was doing. she really did not want us to say things as they were. In another care home, the three ladies who were interviewed by CQC agents were subjected to strong criticism for not lying or for not sugar-coating the truth and facts during their interview and they were blamed for some bad /unfavourable things written in the report by the CQC agents.

Inaccurate Press Reports of CQC

CQC reports should not be made public until the care home has been forcefully closed which usually happens after they have had the opportunity to fix their mistakes/shortcomings or if it is completely unfixable. I have read many newspaper reports following the CQC report and I have noticed that the press is completely not factual. In most cases, they fail to report anything good and solely report everything bad. The press are scavengers who want to attract as many readers as possible for profit which is probably why they report only the bad sides of the CQC reports. This promotes utter condemnation and public shaming of the care homes and sometimes the workers despite the fact that the press report is biased and the fact that the public interest plus objectives of the CQC is to get the care home to make the needed improvements. If the CQC does not support public shaming or trying to close the care home using what is called, 'trial by media, then they should stop the press interfering biasedly. CQC should ban any press retelling of their reports or move to regulate the press to only notify or/and refer their readers to go to the CQC website and read any report in full instead of reporting in a severely biased manner.

Avoid unnecessary interference during inspection

Yes, I agree they visited our Care Home for a necessary duty. They did something bad at one time during their visit. It was dinner time and I was feeding a resident in the dining area. All other Carers were busy too. Suddenly, an upstairs toilet call bell began to ring. I had to pause the feeding to respond as the bell continued ringing. I walked from the dining room on the ground floor to the toilet on the first floor and it was the Local Safeguarding woman who had pressed it. They saw me coming and cancelled the bell. I walked into the toilet and pressed the bell so it started ringing again, I then turned around and asked the two of them, 'who pressed that bell?', gave them a bad look, cancelled the bell and returned to the dining room and continued what I was doing before being interrupted. My reason for including this event in this Memoir is because I felt very sad when it happened because they should not have interrupted a resident's meal time for whatever reason and the call bell should not be pressed recklessly by someone who is not our care home resident. That sort of interference is not part of their job. Even if they needed to check how long it takes us to respond to call bells, they chose the wrong time.

NHS Incontinent team's unsafe orders

Carers should not be given such orders that put them in situations where they cannot do anything right and must make a choice of which bad deed is lesser. For example, the incontinence team ordered that Carers save all incontinent pad of residents under assessment in the building for the incontinence team to be sure, this practice is totally against everything they have been taught about infection control. So, a health-related decision in the sense of bad hygiene or bad infection control if they save pads vs an economic related decision of not strictly avoiding waste or not complying with instructions that may aid the building of trust between the care team and the county's incontinence team. Whatever the Carers do, they are wrong. One bad position to be.

DBS and new Carers

The DBS is very important but the fact that it takes four weeks and that new Carers who are seeking jobs are required to pay up to £62 pounds for enhanced DBS makes it unfair. The four weeks (usually two and a half weeks) of sitting in the house waiting for the DBS is enough to put new Carers off, remember time is money and four weeks of work could be worth over a thousand pounds. In the end, new Carers who wish to venture into the health care sector would begin by losing at least £1000 pounds (time spent waiting for DBS) and another £62 pounds (payment for DBS) before they even start working. There should be a faster way of getting the standard and enhanced checks done in a quicker way and without any costs to the poor Carer seeking a job. The DBS is introduced to boost efficiency in the system, but it has now become a stumbling block for new Carers. This is because experienced Carers looking for a new job or to change job do put in their CV that they have a DBS certificate and are already subscribed to the DBS update service and managers often prefer them to new Carers who do not have a DBS certificate which takes between 4 to 8 weeks and are not already subscribed to the DBS update service. The system should be redesigned to remove this unfair disadvantage. To reduce this 4 to 8 weeks waiting time, new Carers prior to applying to care homes for

194

work should be able to go directly to the government's DBS application webpage, upload their details and have the checks done for free if possible so that their employers can pay at a later date to access the Carer's DBS certificate or have a copy posted to their HR. This will save time and remove the unfair disadvantage.

Closing a care home

Local councils' safeguarding team, who are responsible for assessing care homes and closing those with severe safety issues must ensure all Carers get psychological, financial and needed support to find a new job and to receive their last wages from their employers whose Care Home is being closed. The fact that the employment tribunal charges almost a Carer's monthly wage to get filed is disgusting. It prevents Carers from seeking justice. But it is a bad system to give good benefits to unemployed people, but charge employed people on lowest income over £700 to make employment tribunal claims should they get maltreated by employers.

Mental capacity act clarity about resident's risk-taking

The mental capacity act holds Carers responsible for 'duty of care' to protect people from danger. For instance, If a resident who has no deprivation of liberty authorisation in-place wishes to take a walk through the park at 2:00am risking attack by dangerous animals or risk climbing the stairs and Carers are fully confident that he would fall and such fall might be fatal, their duty of care compels them to stop him and at the same time, the mental capacity act compels them to respect his wishes to take risks and it is against the law to stop him (restricting his freedom). Different trainers give different answers and the extent of unclarity is very significant. It now appears to look like deliberate placing Carers in the middle and in such a dilemma that they get blamed whenever something goes wrong horribly.

References

Alzheimer's Society. (2018). The later stages of dementia (4. Memory). Available: https://www.alzheimers.org.uk/info/20073/how_dementia_pr ogresses/103/the_later_stages_of_dementia/4. Last accessed 17th Mar 2018.

BBC News. (2019). Southampton General Hospital security staff vote for strike. Available: https://www.bbc.co.uk/news/amp/uk-england-hampshire-47636769. Last accessed 17 April 2019.

BBC News. (2019). UK heatwave: Second hottest day on record leads to travel chaos. Available: https://www.bbc.co.uk/news/uk-49106092. Last accessed 26th Jul 2019.

Blanchard, B. (2013). The Law of Compassion. Available: http://beverlyblanchard.blogspot.com/2013/09/the-law-of-compassion.html?m=1. Last accessed 27th April 2019.

Cambridge Advanced Learner's Dictionary & Thesaurus. (2017). scorched-earth policy. Available: https://dictionary.cambridge.org/dictionary/english/scorched-earth-policy. Last accessed 27th Feb 2018.

Department of Education (Education Authority). (2011). Guidance on the commitment to reduce primary class sizes to a maximum of 30 pupils, for pupils at Foundation Stage and Key Stage 1 (Primary 1 to Primary 4), and class sizes in practical subjects. Available: https://www.educationni.gov.uk/articles/pupils-and-classes. Last accessed 17th Mar 2018.

Gillett, F. (28 December 2017). NHS hospitals make a record £174m from car parking... and four of the top 10 most expensive are in London. Available: https://www.standard.co.uk/news/uk/nhs-hospitals-make-a-record-174m-from-car-parking-and-four-of-the-top-10-most-expensive-are-in-a3727961.html. Last accessed 30th Dec 2017.

Halliday, J. (1 Dec 2017). Carl Sargeant: hundreds turn out for former Welsh minister's funeral. Available: https://www.theguardian.com/uk-news/2017/dec/01/carl-sargeant-hundreds-turn-out-former-welsh-labour-ministers-funeral. Last accessed 16th Dec 2017.

Halliday, J. (14 Jun 2017). 'Stay put' safety advice to come under scrutiny after Grenfell Tower fire. Available: https://www.theguardian.com/uk-news/2017/jun/14/stay-put-safety-advice-under-scrutiny-grenfell-tower-fire. Last accessed 28th Feb 2018.

ITV4. (2018). Out of Their Skin (Series 1 - Episode 1 ITV4. 27 November, 22:00). Available: https://www.itv.com/hub/out-of-their-skin/2a5475a0001. Last accessed 29th November 2018.

ITV Report. (8 February 2017). Teachers using body-cams in trial to combat unruly pupils. Available: http://www.itv.com/news/2017-02-08/teachers-using-body-cams-in-trial-to-combat-unruly-pupils/. Last accessed 8th Feb 2017.

ITV Report. (18 July 2018). Exclusive: Sir Cliff Richard says 'if heads roll at the BBC it will be deserved' after he wins privacy case. Available: http://www.itv.com/news/2018-07-18/cliff-richard-bbc-privacy-case. Last accessed 19th Jul 2018.

Morse, A. KCB (Comptroller and Auditor General). (8 February 2018). The adult social care workforce in England. Available: https://www.nao.org.uk/wp-content/uploads/2018/02/The-adult-social-care-workforce-in-England.pdf. Last accessed 26th Feb 2018.

NASUWT-The Teachers' Union. (2019). Physical violence against teachers is a weekly occurrence. Available: https://www.nasuwt.org.uk/article-listing/violence-against-teachers-weekly-occurrence.html. Last accessed 19 April 2019.

National Care Forum NCF. (25 April 2016). Dementia care and LGBT communities: A good practice paper. Available: http://www.nationalcareforum.org.uk/documentLibraryDownl oad.asp?documentID=1228. Last accessed 4th April 2018.

NHS England. (2019). heatwave SUPPORTING VULNERABLE PEOPLE BEFORE AND DURING A HEATWAVE Advice for care home managers and staff. Available: https://www.nhs.uk/Livewell/Summerhealth/Documents/He atwave%2520for%2520care%2520home%2520staff.pdf&ved= 2ahUKEwiUkM2CxJ7iAhVaUhUIHRxzBtkQFjAMegQIBBAC &usg=AOvVaw1Ai8FulF_zmyrriFLOScu2&cshid=155797633 71. Last accessed 17th May 2019.

O'Malley, K. (2019). ROXANNE PALLETT TOLD SHE WAS 'MORE HATED THAN A MURDERER' AFTER CELEBRITY BIG BROTHER 'PUNCH' ROW. Available: https://www.independent.co.uk/life-style/women/roxanne-pallett-celebrity-big-brother-ryan-thomas-punch-reaction-a8952561.html. Last accessed 14th June 2019.

Public HEALTH England (PHE) and National Health Service (NHS). (2019). Every Mind Matters. Available: https:/www.nhs.uk/oneyou/about-one-you/. Last accessed 8th October 2019.

Rayner, G., Edgar, J. and Dixon, H. (29 Apr 2014). Leeds teacher murder: Ann Maguire 'stabbed in the back' in front of 30 pupils. Available: https://www.telegraph.co.uk/news/uknews/crime/10794472/Teacher-Anne-Maguire-was-stabbed-in-back-in-front-of-class-at-Leeds-school.html. Last accessed 8th Feb 2017.

Semlyen, J. (26 September 2016). Dementia and the lesbian, gay, bisexual and trans (LGBT) population. Available: https://www.dementiaaction.org.uk/news/19643_dementia_and_the_lesbian_gay_bisexual_and_trans_lgbt_population. Last accessed 26th Jan 2018.

Snaith, E. (21 April 2019). Two arrested after horse collapses in Cardiff as Easter heatwave grips city. Available: https://www.independent.co.uk/news/uk/home-news/horse-collapses-men-arrested-easter-heatwave-cardiff-city-centre-a8880091.html. Last accessed 22 April 2019.

Syal, R. (7 Dec 2015). Lord Janner found unfit to stand trial for alleged sex offences. Available: https://www.theguardian.com/uk-news/2015/dec/07/lord-janner-found-unfit-stand-trial-alleged-sex-offences. Last accessed 17th Mar 2018.

The Guardian. (2015). Sign of the times of racism in England that was all too familiar. Available: https://www.theguardian.com/world/2015/oct/22/sign-of-the-times-of-racism-in-england-that-was-all-too-familiar. Last accessed 17th Mar 2018.

Thompson, A. (28th October 2015). Care home 'locked down' as police launch murder probe. Available: https://www.leicestermercury.co.uk/news/leicester-news/care-home-locked-down-detectives-667938. Last accessed 8th Feb 2018.

United Nations. (1948). Universal Declaration of Human Rights (UDHR). Available: http://www.un.org/en/universal-declaration-human-rights/. Last accessed 18th Feb 2018.

Wright, S. (28th October 2015). Teacher Vincent Uzomah stabbed at Bradford Dixons Kings Academy offers to help teenager who nearly killed him. Available: http://www.thetelegraphandargus.co.uk/news/13900555.Teacher_Vincent_Uzomah_stabbed_at_Bradford_Dixons_Kings_Academy_offers_to_help_teenager_who_nearly_killed_him/. Last accessed 8th Feb 2017.

Young, S. (27 October 2017). Stop using toilet paper and use wet wipes instead, say Doctors. Available:

https://www.independent.co.uk/life-style/toilet-paper-stop-use-wet-wipes-doctor-health-problems-bidets-a8028906.html. Last accessed 30th Mar 2018.

Printed in Great Britain
by Amazon

55979545R00122